Praise for Bio-Kinetic Testing For Health . .

"Bio-Kinetics helped me where 3 physi
— *Jed Pit*
Blue Cr

*"I felt like I had never been the same since I contracted pneumonia
in December of 1995. I went for Bio-Kinetic testing.
She picked up on everyone of my problems, and knew their causes
without me saying anything about any of them.
She put me on special cleansing diets, and gave me various herbs,
and now I feel as good as new—better, because now I know how to
listen to my body, and how to take care of myself."*
— *Allison Hanna, High School Student*

*"My life is returned! I've taken a seminar on Bio-Kinetic testing
and learned the skill. Even though I am a registered nurse, I feel
like someone has put a diamond in my lap and I treasure this new
found knowledge. It is invaluable."*
— *Michelle Christensen*
Mother, Registered Nurse

*"Our seven year old daughter was having a lot of allergy problems.
We were concerned about her continued dependence on medicine,
so we took her for Bio-Kinetic testing. She is now 12 years old and
with the help of herbs she no longer gets infection in her sinuses."*
— *Toni Rosander, Mother & John (Rosey)*
Rosander, Recreational Director

*"Bio-Kinetic testing and herbs have remarkably improved the
health of my family over the past few years.*
— *Ursula Witzel, Mother*

*"For the first time in years I had energy, my heart functioned
better, and I could go walking."*
— *Janis Jackson, Mother*

"Without knowing anything about him, Bio-Kinetic testing accurately detected that he had a heart murmur and some emotional problems."

> — *Dilleen Marsh, School Teacher*

"I was 22 years old when I started getting migraines. A few months later I started passing out.
I spent four months, several tests, and a lot of money on medical doctors who could not confirm a solid diagnosis.
Through Bio-Kinetic testing, taking herbs and changing my diet, within a month I was completely healthy."

> — *Cindy Nissalke, Mother*

"I cannot begin to calculate the time and money Bio-Kinetics has saved me. It is so exciting to me to have more control over my own health and the health of my family."

> — *Kim Cottrell, Mother*

"Through Bio-Kinetic testing I found the right diet and supplements I needed to promote healing. What a joy it is to feel good again."

> — *Dora Tesch., Mother*
> *Health and Nutritional Counselor*

"I am from a strong scientific background. My dad and uncles are all engineers, scientists, and physicians. I have found Bio-Kinetics to have an unmatched level in diagnosing and treating illness. It has been instrumental in restoring my health and has given me a new life and future wherein I can enjoy being a wife and mom."

> — *Julie Skalla, Mother*
> *BA of Political Science*

BIO-KINETIC TESTING FOR HEALTH

How To Take The Guesswork Out Of Healing

Tisha Mecham

Living Dreams, LLC

Living Dreams, LLC
P.O. Box 313
Sandy, UT 84091-0313
Phone: 801-523-0890
email: tisha@aros.net

Cover & Text Illustrations: Wendy Froshay
Cover Design: Barney McKay Design
Typesetting: Mel Broberg

Manufactured in the United States of America

ISBN 0-9666409-0-X

Dedication

This book is dedicated to my hero, my teacher, my first love
and my strength through childhood storms,
who became my friend and advisor

Glenn L Sorensen

Thank you, dad, for being humble enough
to admit you were not perfect and yet perfect enough
for nine children to follow and to love.

Acknowledgments

- *David Mecham, my husband and partner, who is a man of integrity and strength.*

- *Our children, Rachel, David, Michael, Nathan, Anthon, Lamanda, Newel, Jessica, Tressa, Preston and Maureen, who are the most beautiful people in my life.*

- *My sisters, Loretta, Sheila and Regina, who have always acknowledged and encouraged my gift.*

- *Raland J Brunson, who held my hand and gave me faith to live my dreams.*

- *Wendy Froshay whose art work graces the cover and pages of this book. After countless hours at her easel, she shares her incredible talent and art with you.*

- *Stac'ey Adams whose editing and vision of this book have been an invaluable tool in getting the finished product to the market.*

- *All who have touched my life as I have learned about and used this priceless skill.*

Foreword

On a sunny Autumn day in 1997 I apprehensively rang Tisha Mecham's doorbell. For months, close to a year now, I had been filled with an anger which had an increasingly insatiable appetite, along with what the Dr.'s discovered as a cancerous situation in my female organs, headaches that never went away, a depression that loomed darkly overhead, an energy level that was static, and an overall feeling of misery.

I knew life could and should be better than this. Doing all I knew how to do, counseling with several Dr.'s, using several alternative approaches I still came up empty handed. I was discouraged.

That's when a friend of mine, in fact, the artist and illustrator of this book, Wendy Froshay told me about how Tisha had helped her and her family.

I was skeptical. I didn't know what to expect as it sounded pretty hokey to me. I couldn't understand how someone who didn't know me and only used my swinging feet, cradled in her palms, could tell me how to alleviate or eradicate my pain and discomfort.

When Tisha asked me, no told me, I had been in a serious car accident when I was 6, that's when I knew there was something to this Bio-Kinetic testing that made it stand apart from everything else.

You see, coming home from vacation, 10 days after celebrating my 7th birthday in 1965, my family was involved in a serious 2 car accident which left my mother paralyzed.

Now I'm not saying this testing method is clairvoyant.....what I am saying is, that in this situation, it got my attention. I decided I would follow her suggestions......besides, what did I have to lose. If it didn't work, I'd be no worse off. If it did, well, that thought gave me hope.

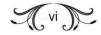

Come to find out I was full of the Epstein-Barr virus, yeast, allergies, some bacteria, my pituitary gland was crooked, my thyroid underactive, my liver full of medicine and my brain and nervous system were under a great deal of stress.

Tisha prescribed a course of action. I followed it to the T. In two weeks when I returned, most of the Epstein-Barr was gone, the yeast was going, she straightened my pituitary gland, reset my thymus and gave me a new direction to go: one accurately designed for me and my system.

Today I'm feeling more alive than I've ever felt. I look forward to feeling even better and obtaining health, wellness and fitness goals I gave up on years ago.

I've even learned how to test myself. This piece of knowledge has given me an indescribable sense of control and freedom. I now feel like I know what to do over the stewardship I've been given regarding my body.

A neighbor of mine has recently been extremely sick. Knowing what I know, with him being open-minded, I shared this skill with him. Through the encouragement and the support of Tisha, a plan was devised to aid him in the relief of his problems. As I walked home, I felt a sense of satisfaction I've never known before. Four days later, the pain had subsided and he was looking to get well and is encouraged to keep doing this designed plan for him, which is bringing such relief.

If you want to gain back control of your life back where it belongs; with you—

If you want peace of mind because you know the exact source of your problems—

If you want to save countless hours of illness or waiting in Dr.'s offices—

If you want to have more money for the fun things in life instead of spending it on Dr.'s and medicines and tests and hospitals —- (Mind you, herbs do cost also. Once you get established, though, they're a lot cheaper than most of the prescriptions out there on the market.....and a whole lot safer for your body.)

If you want to know exactly what you can do to achieve a healthy physical, mental, emotional, and spiritual balance for you—

If you want to know when to seek medical help and when it's something you can take care of yourself—

If you want to spend money only on the supplements and products that are good for your chemically unique body—

If you want to set yourself free from all the confusion regarding the popular health trends out there—

Then learn Bio-Kinetic testing. It will give you the freedom to fly and soar higher in the realms of feeling good than you ever thought possible.

I strongly believe every home would benefit from having this knowledge around.

Victor Hugo said it best in this poem:

Wings

Be like the bird
That, pausing in her flight
Awhile on boughs too slight,
Feels them give way
Beneath her and yet sings,
Knowing that she hath wings.

Thank you, Tisha, for my wings . . .

Here's to you getting yours . . .

Stac'ey Adams

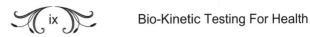

Table of Contents

CHAPTER 1

CHAPTER 2

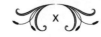

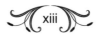

CHAPTER 7

CHAPTER 8

CHAPTER 9

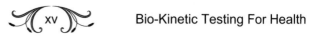

CHAPTER 10

CHAPTER 11

CHAPTER 12

CHAPTER 13

CHAPTER 14

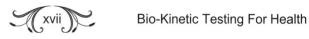
CHAPTER 15

CHAPTER 16

CHAPTER 17

CHAPTER 18

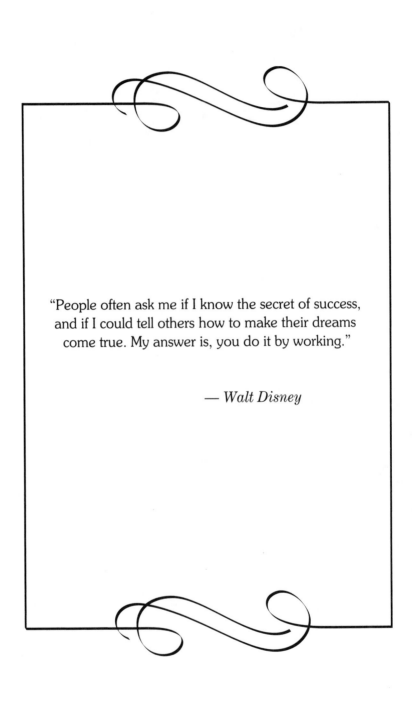

"People often ask me if I know the secret of success, and if I could tell others how to make their dreams come true. My answer is, you do it by working."

— *Walt Disney*

About The Author

Tisha Mecham is a native of Idaho. During her early years she spent much time on the family farm getting to know herself and developing a closeness to nature that would prepare her for the responsibilities of the years to come.

Tisha attended nurse's training after graduation from high school. During this time she discerned a keen aptitude for comforting the sick and afflicted along with a desire to ease human suffering.

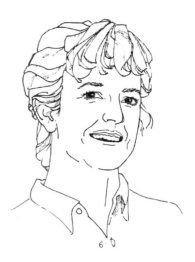

Tisha Mecham

Poor health after a car accident several years later turned her down the path of herbal medicine. This complemented her earlier training as a nurse. As a Master Herbalist, she has seen healing in both the field of medicine and complimentary medicine and has learned to combine them gracefully.

Tisha has counseled both family and friends for many years in nutrition, vitamins and herbs and is highly sought after as a healer. She has written a manual *Bio-Kinetic Testing for Health* and over the years, Tisha has taught classes and seminars where many have come to learn the skills she eagerly shares with them about how to test for health.

Tisha and David are the parents of eleven children. She considers this to be her greatest accomplishment.

Introduction

Several years ago I picked up a book about complimentary medicine that started me on a journey of untold magnitude.

If this is the first book of its kind you have read, I hope to make it as interesting and understandable as possible so you can share the beautiful truths about healing and health that have come to mean so much to me.

This knowledge has come to me through the years in bits and pieces of information as I was ready for it. It is now combined into a self-help guide that will be of benefit to you, the reader, as well as those in your circle of life who may need help at this time.

By reading this book, it shows that you have an interest in your own personal health and that you are one of many who has come to the conclusion that there are powerful alternative methods to healing.

This book will only be the beginning. As you continue to read and study and implement those things that are "truth" to you, you will find the answers you seek.

Tisha :)

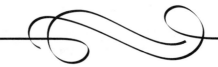

"Life's a pretty precious and wonderful thing.
You can't sit down and let it lap around you . . .
you have to plunge into it;
you have to dive through it!
And you can't save it,
you can't store it up;
you can't horde it in a vault.
You've got to taste it;
you've got to use it.
The more you use, the more you have . . .
that's the miracle of it!"

— *Kyle Chrichton*

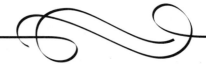

CHAPTER 1

My Story

The question I hear the most is, "How did you get into this?" To understand my heart, motives and actions, you need to know my background.

My life on earth started in June of 1945, which is the year World War II ended. My mother often joked, "You were born when the peace treaty was signed and maybe that is why you are so peaceful." It depends on who you ask whether I was peaceful or not!

I am the second oldest of nine children. We were raised on a farm in Idaho. Farming goes hand in hand with hard work and long hours. If I had known then what I know now, I probably would have appreciated it more.

It was a good life. I rode horses, milked cows, drove tractors, trucks and farm equipment, and had the great outdoors for my schoolmaster.

One day when I was out in the fields with my dad, he picked up some dirt and said, "Farmers

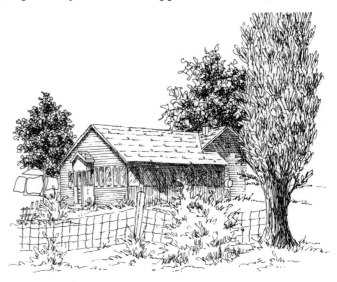

Farm home of my growing up years in Idaho.

work closer with the earth than anyone else. It gets in our blood. We look forward to the first blade of wheat sprouting in the spring and follow it through to the harvest. Every year it is the same. We may have a bad harvest in the fall, but come spring we forget the past year and look forward to a successful new year."

Children request certain things that are family treasures as their parents grow older and get closer to passing on to the next life. If it were possible to request personality traits for an inheritance, I would ask for my dad's sense of humor and optimism. I value those gifts above anything earthly he could leave me.

After graduation from high school, I went to a private Catholic hospital in Idaho Falls, Idaho, where I was trained as a Licensed Practical Nurse. This is where the ideas of healing and helping the suffering became a reality.

The nursing profession was a great experience. I worked at it until our first baby was born. At that time I gave up my license to become a full-time mom. Little did I know that with eleven children in store for me through the years the nursing background I had would never be put aside! In fact, it has been invaluable in raising those children.

The nurses training also prepared me for what was to come in my own personal life.

In 1976 we were living in Texas. One day, riding home from a meeting with some neighbors, we were involved in a car accident. That accident changed the whole course of my life.

There seemed to be no serious injuries at the time. I suffered a whiplash, hit my cheek on a window and was bounced around in the seat.

A few weeks later I began to feel numbness in my arms and lost a lot of strength in them. My hands were so weak I could not pull my baby's shoes on his feet.

A friend suggested I see a chiropractor. Given my earlier training and philosophy, I discounted that idea immediately.

Eventually, however, I gave in. "It can't hurt," I thought. I walked out of his office a different person. Since then I have wondered why there is such a gulf between medical doctors and chiropractors, they both have so much to offer in their own areas of expertise.

I only regret I waited so long to get adjusted because by then my bones and muscles had decided they liked being "out of alignment".

Shortly after the accident and before going to see the chiropractor, I developed a severe pain in my right side just below the rib cage. One night when I laid down in bed, I came right up with a jerk because the pain took my breath away.

The next day I called a doctor, who got me right in. He prescribed a medicine for what he thought was gallbladder problems.

I took one dose of the medicine and began to feel "funny." I had a dry throat and dizziness. I should have recognized what was happening because I had seen allergic reactions to medicine many times during my nursing career.

I can't remember if I took two doses or just one, but the important thing to note here is it can be fatal to take even one dose of the wrong medicine!

By bedtime I was feeling nauseated and cold and achy and thirsty and - well, you name it, I felt it.

When I laid down in bed this time, I felt like I was sinking away into a dark chasm. I had to open my eyes and shake my head to keep myself awake.

I began having visions of my life and saw and understood the choices I had made and the impact they would have on me now. I fought the idea of passing on to the next life because I wanted more time to change some of those things.

I was very thirsty and sat up in bed. Even though I felt dizzy, I struggled to my feet and went to the kitchen where I drank a huge glass of juice.

Feeling somewhat comforted, I started back to the bedroom. I did not get far before I collapsed to the floor.

As I hit the floor, my spirit lifted from my body.

I was in a tunnel with a spiral look to it and was being pulled through at a rapid pace. I could hear what seemed like wind blowing past my ears.

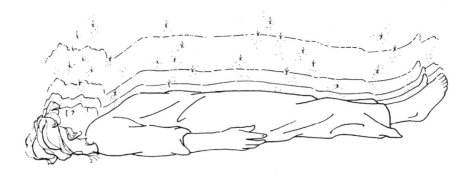

Spirit leaves body

At the end of the tunnel was a wonderful, warm, bright light. I was being drawn towards it. It felt so perfect and so right that I had no fear or anxiety. It was a feeling of absolute peace and joyous anticipation.

About halfway to the Light, it was as if someone put up a hand, stopped me and asked, "Do you want to continue or do you want to go back?"

I can tell you, having left what I had just left - a body racked with pain and nausea, it was a difficult decision. "Out of my body", I felt a warmth, perfection, euphoria and joy that was indescribable. Why would I want to go back?

Then, I remembered my five little children. Would I go back to what I had just left for them? Yes.

The minute I made that decision, my spirit hit my body with a thud. I was sick and miserable, but I was back. My husband was kneeling at my side. Every time he attempted to leave, I felt myself sinking again. I needed physical contact at all times or I would have readily gone back to the spiritual realm.

He wanted to call the ambulance and needed to get dressed, so he went to our oldest daughter's bedroom and brought her to sit beside me. Our little

five-year-old was hardly able to stay awake but did so as her father told her to "talk to Mommy and don't let go of her hand."

I spent the night in the hospital. Tests showed there was "nothing wrong" with me. I was sent home much wiser for the experience.

The feeling that "I could have let go and gone to the next world any minute if I wanted to" lasted for about two weeks. Knowing what I know now, I understand that it takes that long to get an allergen out of the system.

Some profound lessons came from that experience. The one that stood out the most was the constant impression in my mind that if I wanted to get well and stay well, I needed to take charge of my own destiny and not put my life in someone else's hands!

I did not realize at that time where this emphasis would lead. Through the years it has evolved into this very book you are reading. This method of testing will give you the right to take responsibility for your own health and the health of your family.

I opened up my mind to complimentary medicine and went to see the chiropractor. Since that time I have studied herbs, vitamins, stress management, touch for health, acupressure, meditation and visualization, nutrition, earth and energy, and various healing arts.

The things I have learned have been enlightening. I continue to learn and am a different person than I was before the car accident—for the better.

My children have had a much healthier life than I had as a child. It is a joy to see them grow and learn the things I wish I had known at their ages about nutrition and healing.

BIO-KINETIC TESTING

I call my method of testing "Bio-Kinetics". "Bio" is the scientific term for life or living; "kinetics" stands for movement or motion. Simply stated, it is identifying physical signals via the body's electrical energy flow.

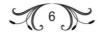

Kinesiology is one of the forms of testing used by chiropractors and others to determine the strength or weakness of a body organ by exerting pressure against an arm or a leg.

When I used kinesiology to test my children I wondered if their muscle was weak because of the constant resistance against it, or if there really was a weakness in their body. I was always looking for a better method.

I continued using what knowledge and skill I had until about five years after the car accident in Texas. We were living in Utah at the time when my sister told me about a woman in Oregon who had a gift of healing. "You should come right up with your eight children and see her!", Sheila said.

Right! Drive for eight hours with a van full of children.

Every parent who knows where every rest stop is between two given destinies knows what I am talking about!

The opportunity to make the trip came a year or so later. When I saw her test my children by using their feet I knew that was the reason I went.

She did not teach me what she was doing, but with the knowledge I already had of kinesiology, body organs, vitamins and herbs, I was able to master the testing with practice and prayer.

What I do may be very different from what she did, but it works and is a unique system that I have never seen anyone else use.

I have worked with Kinesiology, and iridology, and have found this method of testing to be more exact. It takes the guess work out of nutritional supplementation.

Instead of opening the cupboards and indiscriminately passing out vitamins or herbs to our children, we can now test for exact amounts and what and when to give them.

What a thrill you will have as you participate in and decide the right health course for yourself and your loved ones.

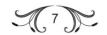

All methods of healing are beneficial. Bio-Kinetics serves to unite them into one method that benefits all. It is the net that catches the healing arts and holds them together.

Not only do I feel comfortable with testing my own loved ones, but it has put me in a position to be able to help others who have come to me seeking help with health problems. I know and understand their quest because I was there not too long ago myself.

Jesus Christ is the source of healing and instruction. Without Divine intervention we would all be lost. When there is no one else to turn to, answers will come to you through inspiration and prayer. I have learned more from my Master Teacher than from any book or class I have attended.

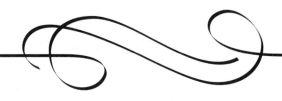

"It is part of the cure to want to be cured."

> *— Seneca*

"When it comes to your health, I recommend frequent doses of that rare commodity among Americans—common sense.

We are rapidly becoming a land of hypo-chondriacs, from the ulcer-and-martini executives in the big city to the patent medicine patrons in the sulphur-and-molasses belt."

> *— Dr. Vincent Askey*
> *former president of the AMA*

"The very success of medicine in a material way may now threaten the soul of medicine. Medicine is something more than the cold mechanical application of science to human disease. Medicine is a healing art. It must deal with individuals, their fears, their hopes, and their sorrows. It must reach back further than a disease that the patient may have to those physical and emotional environmental factors which condition the individual for the reception of disease."

> *— Dr. Walter Martin, another*
> *former AMA president*

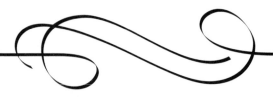

CHAPTER 2

The Healing Path

It has been a rich opportunity to learn about complimentary medicine. One of the most interesting things I have discovered is that there are energies on this earth that affect all that dwell upon it.

What are these energies? They are the electrical powers that control the earth. Gravitational pull is an energy; solar power is another; the ocean, the winds and the rivers have incredible energy; there are beta waves and gamma waves along with others that fill the air.

An energy less understood but just as powerful is the energy of the human body. This energy will be referred to later in the book as you begin to use it in Bio-Kinetic testing.

Every thing endowed with energy has both a negative and a positive pole, which gives balance to it's existence. Consider the magnet that both attracts and repels. This is the strength of any energy field and is called the law of opposites.

And so it is with the human body; if there were no opposition within the body, we would die. Opposition is a fundamental principle necessary to sustain life.

Some examples of this are: when you exercise or over exert yourself, the heart rate increases rapidly. When this happens, a chemical is released that opposes the rapid heart beat and slows it down; insulin opposes or balances out the blood sugar level; and free range of motion is possible because muscles oppose each other. While some muscles tighten, others relax which allows body movement.

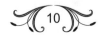

Your personal influence on other individuals is another way of using negative or positive energy.

Radiation

There is one responsibility which no man can evade, that responsibility is his personal influence. Man's unconscious influence is the silent, subtle radiation of his personality—the affect of his words and acts on others. This radiation is tremendous! Every moment of life, man is changing to a degree the life of the whole world.

Every man has an atmosphere which is affecting every other man. He cannot escape for one moment from this radiation of his character, this constant weakening or strengthening of others. Man cannot evade the responsibility by merely saying that it is an unconscious influence.

Man can select the qualities he would permit to be radiated. He can cultivate sweetness, calmness, trust, generosity, truth, justice, loyalty, nobility, and by these qualities he will constantly affect the world.

This radiation to which I refer comes from what a person really is, not from what he pretends to be. Every man, by his mere living, is radiating either sympathy, sorrow, morbidness, cynicism, or happiness and hope—or any of the hundred other qualities.

Life is a state of radiation and absorption. To exist is to be the recipient of radiation. To exist is to radiate.

— David O. McKay

In order to enjoy optimum health, we need to surround ourselves with those things that increase or strengthen our energy. Anything that creates this kind of environment would be called a "positive" as we consider the law of opposites.

Our vital force becomes stronger when we increase in health, understanding, self-confidence, awareness of this earth and our place on it, and when we go forth with a desire to serve others.

Whenever one individual improves in any way, all of mankind benefits. When we raise ourselves to a higher plane of thought or action, there are definite ripples that go out from us to lift others.

When you understand the law of opposites, you also gain a respect for those experiences or individuals who have given you the biggest challenges in your life. It is from facing and overcoming the negative influences in life that you grow and become stronger; or you can choose the opposite path and let the experience weaken you in such a way that you, in turn, become a negative influence in another's life.

During an individual crisis of any kind, try to evaluate the lessons you are learning from this experience, then use these lessons as stepping stones to raise you to a higher plane of thought and action. By so doing, you allow the negative to serve it's purpose, which is to be the catalyst to create a positive strength.

Negative energy may seem to be insurmountable at the time. However, there is something about human nature that seeks after a higher path. In other words, we have more desire to improve our thoughts and look upward and onward than we do to follow the opposite path of gloom and depression.

A positive action will have a lasting effect, whereas a negative experience has a temporary impact. An example of a negative working to create a positive is found in the actions of Mother Teresa of India. She had healing hands and a healing heart. The negative environments of poverty and illness she witnessed created a positive action in her. We will not remember her because of the poverty, but instead she will be remembered for her positive attributes of love and compassion.

If the negative is used as a stepping stone or learning opportunity, we can safely say it will then become a positive experience in the long run.

When we overcome opposition and learn from it we are wiser and stronger. Some of the purposes of life are to gain experience, learn who we are, and what our individual gifts are then use these gifts to benefit others.

Helping another individual find his place on this earth puts both the teacher and the student on a healing path. Anyone who adds to or gives positive direction to another is a healer, no matter what skill they use.

A healing path will bring both negative and positive learning opportunities. These provide the healer with personal insight into the feelings and needs of those who will come seeking help.

In looking back at my life, I see mountains and valleys of events that followed one another that were no accident. They were learning opportunities. I have become what I am today because of them. You, also, are the product of your personal experiences.

This book will be dealing with those things that shape and form a healer's attitude.

The path to healing is not an easy one. Many times you will be required to experience physical, spiritual or emotional setbacks in order to learn how to more fully succor those with whom you will work in the future. Be prepared for that as you seek after the healing gifts.

QUALIFICATIONS OF A HEALER

1. You will need to have insight into all the areas of health: Physical, Emotional, Spiritual, Mental. (These will be explained later.)

2. You need to study about and understand the body—how it is put together and how it functions.

3. Continue to learn all you can about the healing arts. Those could include massage therapy, acupuncture, spinal manipulation, herbs, exercise, foot reflexology, nutrition, homeopathy, cranial work, etc. The more versed you are in the various arts, the more powerful your healing energy becomes.

4. You will begin to develop creative energy. This entails listening to those voices that lead and guide through thought, movement or impression. It also means being able to use creative gifts and move forward without being told everything to do by using your own imagination and visualization.

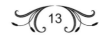

5. You will find yourself overcoming personal weaknesses.
    Jesus Christ said, "Physician, heal thyself." (Luke 4:23, Holy Bible)

6. You will need to have a good personal inner balance. If you are weak
    physically or emotionally, you will tend to take on another's negative
    energy. This is not to say a healer has to be absolutely well all the time, that
    is impossible, but it is important to take an interest in personal care. If a
    cup is full it is able to fill other cups. If it is empty, no one benefits.

7. You will need to ask yourself very often, "What is my intent in learning
    this?"

    Personal intent should be noble. When I ask the participants at my
    seminars why they want to learn this skill, not one ever said they came to
    get rich. They came because they have a desire to help others feel better.
    That is a worthy goal.

    This has become my own personal goal:

    ***To be an instrument in God's hands; to relieve some human
    suffering, and thereby bring a degree of healing and peace to a
    troubled world.***

8. You will need to be a good listener. In order to do so, step outside yourself
    and your own worries to listen to another's sorrows. This will bring comfort
    and cheer to both as you share deep, intense feelings.

9. It is important to feel love. Love is a powerful healing tool. You will need
    to radiate love to those who seek your healing touch.

At this point I would caution you to be sure your feelings towards a client are
always moral and healthy. When someone comes to you in an attitude of
petition and humility, baring his soul, it is so easy to love him. Make sure your
love is Christlike and not one of personal desire. An attitude of lust will surely
lead you astray and begin to diminish the gift of healing.

WHAT IS LOVE?

Love is a much talked and sung about commodity, and lucky is the individual
who possesses it.

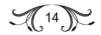

There are as many aspects of love as there are changes of the seasons. Understanding the power of love is part of the path of healing.

Physical love is expressed in the eyes, the hands, the skin, and the close physical contact that binds a couple together. Sexual energy is part of physical love.

Physical love is a desire to meet the physical needs of another. When you go to work to provide a living for, or cook, or clean for, or nurture in illness, or feel physical desires to be with a loved one, you are expressing physical love.

Spiritual love is knowing you have found your soul mate. It is a profound sense of respect and wanting to be around someone because of a special tenderness you share being together. You may find yourself saying, "This time it is different. This love just feels right. I have never felt such a peace with anyone else". This joyous feeling is not necessarily physical, though looking into his eyes can stir a special need to become one in every aspect with your spiritual love.

Emotional love is a love of compassion, empathy, and comfort. It is the warmth of his arm around your shoulder and knowing he is listening to your every word and understanding you with his soul. Emotional love is positive encouragement and words of caring and kindness.

When compliments are bestowed and words of love are spoken, with emotional love you not only hear but can actually feel the truth of the spoken words deep in your heart.

Mental love is being able to talk about ideas and concepts that you both understand and are excited about. It involves setting goals together, encouraging your loved one to excel in mental pursuits or a chosen occupation. Sitting and discussing things of the opera, the world, politics, religion, or any thing where you say, "We are on the same wave length", expresses mental love.

Mental love includes a quiet pride you feel in your loved one. You are aware of his personal accomplishments and appreciate his place in this world.

10. A healer needs to be open-minded. When new ideas are presented, they should be evaluated. I have read some great things, and I have also read things that I refer to as "fluff." It is good to be informed, and on the other hand, be careful not to be pulled off track by unethical ideas. By listening to your inner core, learning to test products (which will be discussed later), and praying earnestly for the best gifts, you will begin to develop a feeling of those things that are truth to you.

11. A keen sense of humor is a great asset. Of course, there is a time to laugh and a time to refrain from laughter, but in most of the daily situations in which we find ourselves, there can be a humorous side.

    I spent two years in Italy as a missionary for my church. During this time I learned a technique that has served me well. At the end of each day, I sat down and wrote the fun, funny, humorous or outlandish experiences of the day. I can read those experiences today and still enjoy the humor.

12. A valued attribute is the spirit of forgiveness. None of us knows what has transpired in the life of individuals to make them behave like they do. Only God knows the intent of the heart. Leave the judgment to Him. Our duty is to be a cheerleader rather than a critic.

13. You will find it fitting to wear a heart of putty and the hide of a rhinoceros. Listen to others and let them know they are loved and understood.

Often, all someone needs is another human being who is willing to sit and listen as he vocalize the feelings of his heart. Simply getting feelings out in the open is healing. When you are listening to others' stories of hurt and agony, imagine those words falling on the floor and disappearing, or floating away into the thin air.

Those were his personal experiences and you do not have to relive them again. Learn from others so that perhaps you will not have to walk the same path some time in your life.

. . . and if you can do all this, then know for sure you have entered the healing realm, my friend.

CAUTIONS

There are a few helpful guidelines to consider before you begin testing.

1.   Never test a child without his parents' permission.

     I had a son who came running in from play and asked, "Mom, will you test Robby? His thumb got jammed!"

     On another occasion I had tested children without their parents being consulted and I found out through hurt feelings and accusations that I was NOT their mother as far as health matters are concerned. Parents should be respected.

     A statement like, "Of course I'll test Robby if he'll call his mom and see if it's okay with her" will alleviate misunderstandings.

2.   Do not let testing replace daily decisions.

     God has blessed each one of us with adequate intelligence to figure out most of life's questions. This testing should not be used to see if it's a good idea to do the shopping, or go to work today, or even get out of bed!

3.   Do not use this to take the place of prayer.

     When you work with this powerful energy long enough, you will come to know God in a special way. We still pray to Him and take questions and needs to Him. Prayer has its place as does the testing.

4.   I have found prayer to be very useful in the development of Bio-Kinetic testing skills.

     In the classes I have taught, some students learn the skill quickly. They take to it like a fish takes to water. It is natural and easy. Others have to work harder at it, but with persistence it does come.

     One of my students attended a seminar with her mother and her sister. They seemed to learn the skill faster in class which discouraged this individual. I could tell when she left that she had feelings of frustration over not being able to test like her family members were able to do.

The next day was Sunday. She took the things she had learned in class to God and prayed all day for an understanding.

Late Sunday night she called to say she felt sick and could she come over for testing. Due to the lateness of the hour, I reminded her that she had learned the skill. I told her to sit in a comfortable chair, hold the phone to her ear and let me walk her through her testing over the phone.

It was exciting when I heard her voice come over the line and exclaim, "It works! It works!" She needed time to think about it, pray about it, and have a reason to use it. All of this happened in one day. Since then, several family members have come to her for testing.

Compare testing skills to musical talents.

I taught piano for several years. Some students had a natural ability in music, but if they did not practice they would be passed up by students who were less skilled but more determined to learn. Those who really wanted to play applied themselves and became amazingly excellent in music.

5. Do not try to see the future or determine the sex of an unborn baby. Bio-Kinetic testing is for here and now, for immediate health things.

6. It is possible to influence the test results with your own mind.

For example: How many parents want their children to be sick? Of course, no one does. So, when you are testing your own child, be open minded in knowing that you now have the skills to help them over come illness. Avoid thinking, "You can't be sick. Please don't be sick. There is nothing wrong with you" ... etc ....

The right kind of a thought would be, "I want to know if there is something going on so we can test for it and decide what needs to be done to help."

7. Never diagnose what you deem to be serious health problems unless you are a qualified health professional.

When I first started working with the public, I had an older gentleman come to me for testing who had a weakness in his heart. This was the first time I had encountered something more serious than just the common cold.

Many thoughts went through my mind. I tried to determine the best way to tell him without diagnosing. Suddenly the thought came to ask him this question: "Have you ever had your heart tested?" He told me he had. Next question, "What did they find?"

At this point he leaned forward and asked, "What do you find?" This put me on the spot. I told him my testing revealed a weakness in the heart muscle on the left side. He slapped his knees and said, "That's exactly what the doctor said." He was on medicine for it.

If your client has not been tested medically for the weakness you find in a particular organ, then question him about symptoms he may be having. Some of these could be gas, cramping, nausea, heart palpitations, headache, dizziness, or whatever that organ feels like when it is out of balance.

When he agrees he experiences these, then tell him what your testing revealed. Unless he is in denial about pain, or has a way of ignoring it, he already knows something is not right.

If there is something wrong that needs medical help, now is the time to encourage him to seek adequate medical attention.

8. Prepare for both negative and positive feedback. More than likely you will receive both.

Not everyone accepts or understands the ways of complimentary medicine.

The evidence of the good you do with this work will be seen in the faces of those who get their lives back and are healthy, happy, and productive.

I heard a story several years ago that may help you understand the pain of criticism or of being misunderstood that many times accompanies this kind of work.

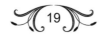

There was a man climbing a mountainside. As he reached up over the top a rattle snake bit his hand.

He was faced with a choice at that time. He could either climb back to his jeep that was at the base of the cliff and get some help, or he could continue to the top, chase down the rattler, and kill it for biting him, which choice would allow the rattlesnake poison to spread throughout his body.

There are many kinds of "rattle snakes" out there who will bite and sting for no provoked reason.

You can choose to let their unkind words or negative criticism get you down, or you can continue to share the knowledge and skills you learn, sharing them for the benefit of those who are interested.

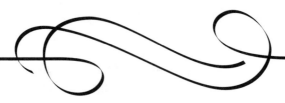

Paul Harvey Speaks Out

Some medical doctors remain unconvinced that vitamin pills are good for anything. Nutrition was mostly ignored in medical education until this recent decade, so it is understandable of some doctors are as unsold on vitamins as some Americans are oversold.

Other doctors would like vitamins to be available only on prescription. They argue that for you to prescribe to yourself may be dangerous. There is no evidence of any widespread misuse. There is, however, a great danger from the misuse of prescription drugs.

A recent eight-year study at 72 poison control centers revealed that sleeping pills and tranquilizers killed 460 people. Analgesics led to 715 deaths. Antidepressants accounted for 805 fatalities. Cardiovascular drugs killed another 360. There were 2,500 people killed by accidental or intentional overdose of drugs. During that same eight years the number of people killed by vitamins was zero. There were no reported fatalities from taking vitamins either by children or adults. Which suggests that vitamins, whatever their benefits, are 2,500 times safer than drugs.

Meanwhile, doctors who do recognize benefits from vitamin therapy are recommending them to overcome high cholesterol, to reduce cancer risk, to prevent or relive many chronic health problems.

— Quoted from The Health Forum
of Utah, July 1993

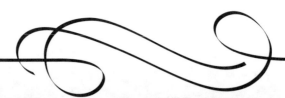

CHAPTER 3

Health: A Personal Choice

How many times have you asked yourself: "Do I need to go see a doctor with this illness or is it just a virus?"

Or, "I wish someone would tell me what to do for my sick child; I feel so helpless."

No matter who we are or where we live, keeping the physical body healthy is a common concern. Many guidelines have been given to us by health care professionals, government, and religious leaders on how to enjoy a healthy lifestyle.

Becoming informed then living what we learn to the best of our knowledge is taking a positive step in the direction of personal health.

There are four main reasons why Bio-Kinetic skills should be learned and lived.

1. Decrease unnecessary lawsuits.

Far too many of us depend on someone else to keep us well. It's time for us to become more responsible for our own health. When we expect someone else to heal us, and they don't, the tendency is to initiate a lawsuit to satisfy what we deem an injustice.

The courts of our land are overloaded with cases of this kind. When responsibility for personal actions comes back and rests upon the shoulders of the individual where it needs to be, we will all be better off.

When I worked as a nurse in the late 1960s and early 1970s, we were allowed to do our job without fear of a lawsuit hanging over our heads. It was a good feeling to be able to give a back rub or even hug a patient if we felt like they needed it.

This kind of bedside manner is rapidly becoming a thing of the past. We have all become losers in the arena of medicine as the battle with lawsuits tears at the very fiber of healing.

2. Increase awareness of preventive health practices.

Doctor James Fletcher, former director of the National Aeronautics and Space Administration (NASA), a scientist on the team that developed the first artificial heart, and former president of the University of Utah, has said many people hang onto bad health habits then rely on doctors to cure them when they are sick.

"It's clear that we need to focus more on prevention of disease and not a cure. How to do this is not clear because doctors and even hospitals are not motivated to do that.

"I don't smoke and I don't drink . . . I kind of resent having to pay all of this money—$1 out of $8 that I earn—into taking care of those people who do have those habits.

"Ultimately we are going to have to deal with that problem because people will revolt against having to pay for the care of people who refuse to take care of their own bodies. Most people don't mind paying for true medical emergencies, but they don't want to pay for those who risk their health against medical and other advice." (Deseret News, November 9, 1990)

3. Decrease medical expense.

When you consider the cost of prescription medicine, it's reason enough to be on guard against what has become a very profitable business in our country.

Prescription drug prices rose three times faster than general inflation in the 1980s.

"Congress needs to do more to curb the increase. While general inflation during the period (1980s) was 58 percent, prescription drug prices rose 152 percent". This information came from a 1991 report released by the Democratic staff of the Senate Special Committee on Aging.

Those who live on a pension or limited income are hardest hit. When my father-in-law needed medicine for a bladder infection, the family paid $5 per pill, which had to be taken three times a day for 10 days. It became quite expensive, and this was out-of-pocket expense.

4. Increase feelings of freedom and peace that come from being a partner in your own personal health care.

Making health a personal choice means not having to rely on prescription medicine except when you feel it is absolutely necessary to preserve life or overcome a stubborn illness.

I decided I would never put medicine in my mouth or in the mouths of my children without first testing to see if there was an allergy to it.

What a gift this would be for doctors to know how to test their patients on a medicine before prescribing it.

In his book, Life after Life, Doctor John Moody interviewed numerous individuals who claim to have had a near-death experience. Of interest to me were the stories that were prompted by a drug reaction.

We are each chemically unique. What may be normal for one person may be toxic to another. We need to know and respect that fact.

An article entitled, "Are Victims of Depression Getting Wrong Drug Dosages?" (Deseret News, August 11, 1991) sheds some light on this subject.

In this article, Dr. Paul J. Orsulak, a professor of psychiatry at the University of Texas Southwest Medical Center in Dallas, says about half of all patients taking antidepressants are given either too little or too much medication.

Further, he says: "Doctors treating patients for depression often depend upon trial and error to establish the right levels of the drugs and many patients fail to respond because they get inadequate doses.

"Doses of antidepressants recommended by pharmaceutical companies are based on average requirements and often give poor results for individual patients."

Based on his studies, Dr. Orsulak found that out of 100 male patients receiving antidepressants, "30 will receive sub-therapeutic levels, 15-20 will get toxic levels, and the rest would receive appropriate levels."

How much easier it would be to test the patient for the exact amount at the time of the visit. Bio-Kinetic skills allow this to happen.

An added bonus comes if doctors become informed about non-prescription products and test for those first. Medicine would then be used only as a back-up or with individuals most chemically compatible with prescription medicine.

You want to be responsible for your own health. Reading this book shows that you are interested in health options. Once you are informed, it is easier to make decisions for yourself and your loved ones. It is your God given right to know what is best for you as an individual.

My hope is that each of us will become informed about our own health needs, know what options are available, and then follow the course that leads to greatest healing and happiness.

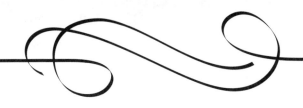

WORDS THAT MATTER

by

Robert Rodale
Late editor of
Prevention Magazine

I am electric. And so are you. And so is
every living cell, every stone, every star.
For, as modern science reveals, the universe
hums with electromagnetism. Electricity
powers suns, kitchen toasters and ticking
hearts. In the natural world, it forms
invisible crisscrossing roadways for migrating
birds, animals and monarch butterflies. It
is, scientists are discovering, a force in the
healing of human wounds. It's everywhere. So
is the electromagnetism of the spirit. By this
I mean the kind of spiritual electricity we feel
when we quicken and renew ourselves with trans-
cending ideals, with a tingling awareness of
beauty in the world, with peace of mind. The
current flows, and we're regenerated. And if
the charge is potent enough, even our bodies
may respond.
— *Prevention Magazine, January 1991*

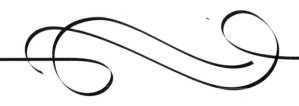

CHAPTER 4

Energy

When we attempt to explain the power of energy, we compare it to going into a room, flipping a light switch and seeing the light go on. We do not see the energy as it goes through the wires, but we see the end result.

This is how it is with Bio-Kinetic testing. You cannot see the energy that runs the testing, but you can see the end result.

There are several forms of energy that affect the human body, and like the electrical charges of magnets, there are both negative and positive pulls.

Science teaches us that the individual body cell generates energy. Each body cell is like a miniature electrical generator with a small "sodium/potassium" pump. As the negative and positive elements move back and forth across the cell membrane, energy is released.

> *"First, potassium ions flow into the cell, reducing the negative charge (depolarization).At a certain point the properties of the membrane change and the cell becomes permeable to sodium, which rapidly enters the cell and causes a net positive charge inside the cell. This is called the action potential . . . the size of the action potential is self-limiting, because a high internal sodium concentration causes the pumping out first of potassium and then of sodium ions, restoring the negative charge in the cell (Repolarization). The whole process takes less than one-thousandth of a second".*

> — *(Funk and Wagnalls Encyclopedia, 1983, Volume 18)*

Through the natural physical processes that go on every second of every day in the human body, energy plays a very important part. This energy has been studied and mapped out by those who have used it for years in their healing arts. An example of this is Oriental Medicine which uses a form of healing called acupuncture. Acupuncture outlines the path of energy in the human body as accurately as a road map is used in driving a car to a given destination.

The energy follows designated paths called meridians. They are located throughout the body and are the transporters of energy. The meridians have been measured by modern electrical technology. With practice, we can learn to feel these meridians (see illustration on opposite page).

There are 14 Meridians that go from the trunk of the body to the hands or feet, from the hands or feet to the trunk, and in a complete circle around the trunk from front to back.

The meridians lie on the surface of the skin and cannot be seen with the naked eye. Along the meridian path are specific acupuncture points. The actual points where needles are inserted are as small as the head of a pin. It takes years of training to be able to locate those points exactly. Modern electrical equipment assists in finding them through the use of sound and lights.

Acupressure and massage therapy are also beneficial to stimulate the acupuncture points. These forms of healing move the energy over a broader area while acupuncture hits the point directly on target.

The Chinese believe that all forces on this earth are moved by and infused with energy, which they call the Chi (Chee). The Chi has two polarizing forces called the yin and yang. In Western Medicine, we call it the negative and positive energy.

Yin is the dark, passive, receptive element of energy (or the negative). Yang is the light, active, giving, positive element.

When the yin and yang are in balance, health is the result. Acupuncture balances the yin and yang.

Another study of this energy deals with what is called the chakra. There are different ideas about how many chakra actually exist.

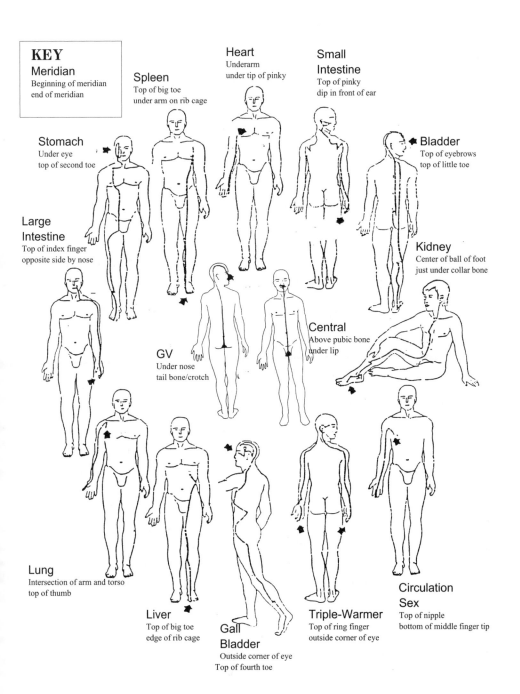

KEY
Meridian
Beginning of meridian
end of meridian

Spleen
Top of big toe
under arm on rib cage

Heart
Underarm
under tip of pinky

Small Intestine
Top of pinky
dip in front of ear

Stomach
Under eye
top of second toe

Bladder
Top of eyebrows
top of little toe

Large Intestine
Top of index finger
opposite side by nose

Kidney
Center of ball of foot
just under collar bone

GV
Under nose
tail bone/crotch

Central
Above pubic bone
under lip

Lung
Intersection of arm and torso
top of thumb

Liver
Top of big toe
edge of rib cage

Gall Bladder
Outside corner of eye
Top of fourth toe

Triple-Warmer
Top of ring finger
outside corner of eye

Circulation Sex
Top of nipple
bottom of middle finger tip

Meridians of the body

The Eastern philosophy believes there are seven chakra, the American Indian believes there are eight, and the Western concept believes in nine. The methods of bringing these chakra into balance vary with the culture. The methods range from meditation, incense burning, sweat baths, circle dances, drumming, prayer, singing, visualization, crystals, and hands on healing.

When you are able to see colors around a person, or the aura, you are looking at the chakra. Each chakra center radiates a different color.

The chakra have pools of energy that lie directly in line with the core of the body. They have been described as whirlwind-like energies spinning in a clockwise position. When they are weakened, they spin backwards, or even become limp. This interferes with the transmission of proper energy needed for balance and health. The attempt is made by different methods to set them spinning strong and in the right direction, thus promoting health at the inner or physical level.

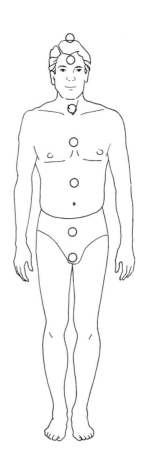

Seven Chakra

The chakra radiate about three feet out from the body in all directions, forming a perfect shield or cocoon of protection to the body.

The chakra could be called the energy pools that draw in energy from the universe, and the fourteen meridians are the transporter of that energy at the physical level.

The chakra are decreased in size by negative forces. These forces mostly come from within, where there is illness, negative thoughts, or unrighteous desires. By the same token, the chakra energy field can be expanded by vibrant health, positive thoughts, and ideas of love and service.

This field can be measured. Here are a couple of techniques to give you an idea.

1. Take some sturdy wire—like clothes hangers. Straighten the hangers, and cut them into equal lengths, between 12"-16". Bend the wires in a perpendicular direction about five to six inches down from the top. Now, holding the wires in both hands, point the bent top towards someone, holding the wires straight ahead.

Let the wires rest in your hands in a lose grip, almost like holding the hand of a small child—firm but gentle. If you hold too tight, the wires cannot move.

As the wires point at an individual, you should concentrate on his energy field and imagine measuring it with the wires. As you do so, the wires will begin to move outward. This gives you an idea of how "wide" or strong that person's energy field is.

Measuring a person's energy field using wires. When the wires are spaced wide, the energy field is strong.

With the wires held lose in your hands and pointed towards the individual, ask him to think of something negative. An example could be of how someone made him mad, or a movie full of violence or sex he may have witnessed.

What has happened to his energy? The wires more than likely will not move outward. Walk towards the individual and try to pick up his energy. You should be able to walk right up to him and the wires will not move outwards, and in fact, they may even cross inwards as a display of negative energy.

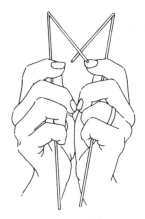

Now, step back about 10 feet and ask the individual to think of someone he loves deeply, or of an especially inspiring or moving experience. An example of this might be attending a musical performance, or

Negative energy displayed.

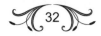
looking at the ocean, or surveying the wonders of the Grand Canyon or other beauties of the world. Ask him to concentrate on how he feels or felt at that time.

What happens to the wires this time? If you are holding them right, the wires will rapidly swing outwards as the energy radiated becomes strong and again fills the room.

2. Another way of detecting energy potential is to stand in front of someone and place your hands on each side of his face. Hold your hands about three to four inches away from his face. Be still and hold your hands in place for a minute or so without touching him. Notice how the heat begins to build up between your hands and his face. When two energies are brought together, the heat or electrical excitement bounces around with more intensity.

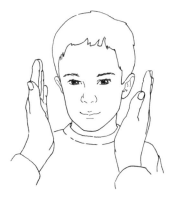

Detecting heat caused by energy build up.

Cameras have been invented that can actually take pictures of the energy flow around living things. These cameras take what is called Kirlian Photography. It is a photograph of the aura of the object.

Ancient artists attempted to draw the energy field that was seen around Jesus Christ. Most pictures of Him show a halo around his head or a bright glow around His whole body.

When Christ is talked about, it is with awe and respect. His energy fills the whole universe.

When we think about the aura of someone, we are thinking about the energy they emit. Some people see the colors of the aura or chakra, some sense it, and some are able to feel it.

As we increase in energy, those around us are strengthened by our positive radiation. This makes for a wonderful home life when all are speaking, thinking, and emitting good energy one to another instead of angers, hatreds,

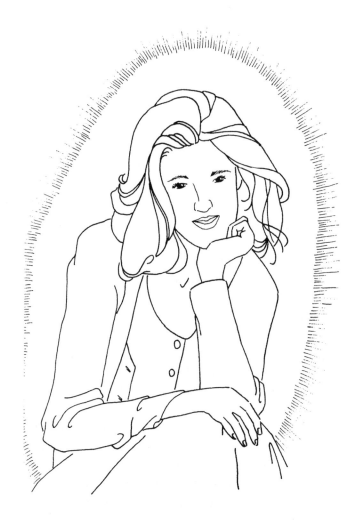

Aura or energy emitted by body.

and fears. When we project positive words, looks, and actions to others, it is returned to us. This elevates the health of everyone in our circle!

Other methods that can be used to increase healing via the energy field are music, colors, humming, massage, ringing bells, poetry, artwork, etc.

I attended a concert one Christmas in which some high school students rang bells to play the music. There were no other instruments, only the bells. As the bells rang, they vibrated the air and blended in such a way that we recognized immediately the songs they were playing.

I thought how much like other healing energies this is. There is a certain "vibration" to herbs, flowers, colors, smells, artwork, and musical pitch. As vibrations from these move through the air, they are recognized by certain body organs and/or the chakra. The vibrations are received into your energy field where they create a healing response within the body.

This works on the same principle as a tuning fork. A trained ear can recognize the pitch of a tuning fork and tune a musical instrument to it. Our chakra are trained to serve us in such a way. The vibration will be different from one individual to another which means we may respond to a color or sound differently than anyone else would. This is why there are many moods to music, different shades of color, forms of art, tastes to food, smells to perfumes, and flowers available for our yards.

As musical instruments vary in pitch and vibration, so our response varies to the energy around us.

Tuning Fork

In the work I have done with colors, I find they also have emotional significance. There are no fast rules on what a color might mean to everyone because we are each unique in our chemical and emotional responses. Where red to one person means pain and anger, to another it may serve to bring bravery and strength into their life.

Many times people wear colors similar to what they subconsciously want to radiate to others, or they wear colors to strengthen an individual weakness. An example of this might be wearing pink on a date to help speak of your love; or, if I were going for a business interview, I would choose to wear green which reduces stress and encourages prosperity.

Wearing a colored stone around the neck will do the same thing. You can either place the stone in a soft bag, or get it made into a necklace to wear around your neck.

Some of the colors and emotions increased by their use are:

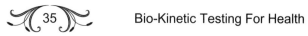

The Color Emotion Table

Color	Intended result
Purple or lavender	Inner peace, calming, inspiration, verbalize feelings, healing heartache, connecting to Spirit.
Pink/Rose	Love, self confidence, eases sexual and emotional imbalance, soothing, relaxing, clears anger, guilt, jealousy, and fears.
Golden brown	Purifies blood, strengthens energy field, connected to God, service, will power, clears perception, helps when going through change.
Green	Balancing, grounding, positive for growth and a new beginning, draws out negative, attracts prosperity, reduces stress, gives inner guidance, aids movement of energy, stands for healing, helper, nurturer, reveals subconscious blocks.
Orange	Stimulates appetite, reduces fatigue, lifts energy, ambition, increases immunity and sexual potency.
Gold/Yellow	Sunshine, clears the mind, gives cheerfulness, hope, self esteem, increases intellect, raises blood pressure, is an anti-depressant.
Blue	Calming, lowers blood pressure, color of teachers, sensitivity, cooling, shielding.
White	Purity, truth, knowledge, peace and comfort, taking away pain.
Red	Stimulates, excites, warms the body, increases heart rate, brain activity, passion, expresses strong feelings of love when mixed with rose, sexual passion when mixed with orange, purging, burning out disease, clear red is moving anger, dark red is stagnant anger.
Black	Promotes a forgetting, or absence of light; to others it gives protection, state of grace, silence and peace.

Chinese Guidelines

Chinese medicine gives certain colors to healthy body organs. Wearing corresponding colors will strengthen these organs, as well as eating certain foods of that particular color.

Liver, eyes = green

Lung, hair = white

Kidney, ears = black

Heart, tongue = red

Spleen, mouth = yellow

Personality Colors

A popular trend from the 1960's was to give a test and determine individual personality strengths through colors. If you fit one of these categories, then perhaps you would feel more comfortable in the corresponding color. Some people fall into more than one category, as personalities are very diverse.

Red = Power, leadership, strong sense of right or wrong.

Blue = Relationships are important, people oriented, loving, caring, good listener.

White = Peacemaker, not strongly opinionated.

Yellow = Just want to have fun, life of the party, liven up the world.

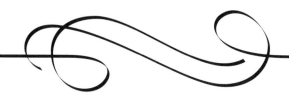

AN INDIAN PRAYER

(Anonymous)

Oh Great Spirit whose voice I hear in the winds,
And whose breath gives life to all the world,
Hear me!
I am small and weak,
I need your strength and wisdom.
Let me walk in beauty, and make my eyes ever behold
the red and purple sunset.
Let my hands respect the things you have made and my ears sharp
to hear your voice.
Make me wise so that I may understand the things you have taught.
Let me learn the lessons you have hidden in every leaf and rock.
I seek strength, not to be greater than my brother,
but to fight my greatest enemy—myself.
Make me always ready to come to you with clean hands and straight eyes.
So when life fades, as the fading sunset,
my spirit may come to you without shame.

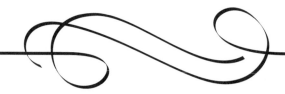

CHAPTER 5

The Total Health Picture

There is a Far East Indian belief that everyone is a house of four rooms: a physical, a mental, an emotional, and a spiritual room. Most of us tend to live in one room most of the time, but unless we go into every room every day, even if only to keep it aired, we are not complete.

Every individual has a favorite room. This is where personal talents and strengths lie. Being in other rooms has to be worked at but can become comfortable with effort.

In order to work with healing, it is important for us to know that health is not just physical. Total health is keeping all four rooms in balance.

Your overall health affects who you are, what you become, and how you act. Making healthy choices and living responsibly ensures a quality lifestyle.

PHYSICAL

The physical aspect of health deals with the actual mechanics of keeping the physical body alive, healthy, and functioning within our capabilities.

There are many things that concern us physically. A few of these are 1) diet, 2) exercise, 3) nutritional supplements, 4) sleep/rest, and 5) size, and weight.

I would like to address each of these individually.

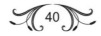

1. Diet

The Food and Drug Administration has developed some dietary guidelines that are very good. The most recent is called the food pyramid. For more information on this and other nutritional guidelines available, see your web site at www.fda.gov.

The pyramid program emphasizes whole grains as a foundation, followed closely with generous servings of fruits and vegetables. The next pyramid level advises milk and milk products with meat servings used sparingly, and finally, fats, oils and sweets used rarely.

FOOD PROCESSING DESTROYS VITAMIN CONTENT

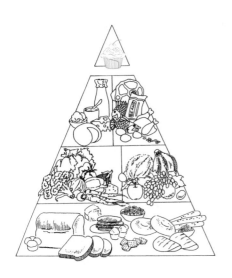

FDA Recommended Food Pyramid

In this day of modern machinery, appliances, and vitamins, have you stopped to ask yourself how you really feel physically? Are you a nervous wreck? Are you overweight or anemic? Do you always have a cold or the flu? Do you suffer from a quick temper, frequent headaches, muscle cramps, mental depression, frequent backaches or constant tooth decay? If so, chances are you have become a victim of poor nutrition brought on by modern-day food processing.

Almost invariably food processing destroys the live food process in our foods. It strips away essential vitamins and minerals, makes our flour and rice white, then adds deadly chemicals, sugars, and bleaches to guarantee a longer shelf life.

Research, study, and personal experience have proven that a lot of our physical ailments today are brought on by improper eating. A wise statement is "natural is better."

There are certain intangible substances in seeds and cells of every living thing that contribute to their growth and sprouting. These substances are called enzymes, and enzymes could be called the live food process.

The human body is a miraculous creation. It has the ability to rebuild itself and thereby overcome most illness and injury. However, to be able to rebuild itself properly from within, it needs to be provided with all the necessary tools or building blocks. These come from the vitamins, minerals, enzymes, and amino acids found in our diet.

Oxygen is one of the most essential elements. As soon as food is cooked, its oxygen is lost. Enzymes are destroyed at 130 degrees F. Consider then the destruction done during commercial food processing. Foods are heated to destroy any live element that might cause spoilage after several weeks on the shelf. This is a strong argument for eating foods as God created them in a pure and natural state.

Along with the failure to nourish the body properly, processed foods aren't able to aid in proper waste elimination. Waste retention is the main cause of a great number of physical ailments.

Norman Walker, D. Sc., who is a member of the National Medical Society, International Society of Naturopathic Physicians, National Association of Naturopathic Herbalists and British National Society of Herbalists, has spent years researching and teaching ways to live a long healthy life. He has written several books dealing with his research. From his book, Become Younger, we learn that "Every organ, limb and part of the body has three important nerve endings, one is in the iris of the eyes, one is in the walls of the colon, and the other is in the sole of the feet."

Iridology, or reading the body's energy through the eyes, makes it possible to see what is going on in any organ of the body. Foot reflexology (massaging the feet) increases nerve flow and healing energy to every body part. Without proper stimulation, the colon becomes sluggish. "When it is clean and normal, we are well and happy. Let it stagnate and every organ of the body becomes poisoned and we age prematurely, look and feel old, and the pleasure of living is gone." (Dr. Walker, Become Younger)

After the sudden death of Elvis Presley, many articles in several magazines and newspapers labeled his diet as one consisting of junk foods. An article

from the Readers Digest, January 1978, p. 75, said that he was overweight and "loved such foods as peanut butter, banana splits, olives and burnt bacon. He suffered from hypertension, an impacted or enlarged colon, mild diabetes, and had a liver problem."

The fibers of raw fruits and vegetables are very much like magnets as they move through the body. They attract waste products and remove them from the system, unlike cooked denatured foods that act more like a mop swabbing through the intestines often leaving a coating of slime.

Along with fresh raw fruits and vegetables, whole grains are recommended.

Wheat has long been known as the staff of life. Early grain millers ground wheat by crushing it between two large stones. No heat was used in the process. This method preserved valuable nutrients.

In the mid 1800s a silk bolting cloth was invented that separated the bran from the flour. Then in 1874 a steel roller mill came along that put the wheat through a rapid process that involved heat.

The wheat germ gummed up the rollers so it was decided that wheat germ had to go. The wheat germ is the life center of the wheat. Wheat sprouts from the germ. Wheat germ is very rich in vitamin E, which is a vital nutrient for the heart.

Coronary heart disease has become one of the major causes of death in our society.

Rice has gone through a similar process. Thiamine (B1) prevents a disease called beriberi. Eighty percent of this vitamin is lost in the processing of turning brown rice into white rice.

When you look at the popular cereals delighted children pack out of the grocery store every day, it is of concern that so many of the cereals are no longer what we could call "whole grains."

From the Journal of Nutrition, Vol. 53, Marguerite A. Constant says, "Many commercial cereals contain more sugar than grain. Nutritional experts have cited experiments where the high carbohydrate in refined white flour, corn flakes, wheat flakes, oatmeal, and white rice products cause tooth decay in

experimental animals." Cereals made with natural grains reduced tooth decay drastically.

This brings up another nutritional giant: Sugar. "Approximately 100 years ago every American consumed about ten pounds of sugar per year. The present figures are horrifying. Up to 200 pounds of sugar are consumed annually by every man, woman and child. Three billion dollars a year are spent for candy." (Horsley, Commercial Foods Exposed)

"The heart is regulated by the amount of carbonic acid in the blood. The more sugar that is eaten, the higher the carbonic acid content, and thus an increase in the heartbeat". (Become Younger, Dr. Norman Walker)

An important step to take in the direction of personal health would be to limit, if not eliminate completely, refined sugars from the diet. A diet that is constantly high in sugar could result in serious heart problems.

Another health concern is the preservatives and additives put in our foods to enhance shelf life.

When you read the label of food boxes it reads like a pharmaceutical page. Some of those products are safe; some are damaging to the body.

These additives could be things like pesticides, certain antibiotic or hormone residue, chemicals from packaging materials, preservatives, stabilizers, emulsifiers, dyes, trace minerals, and synthetic substances.

The best way to avoid those things is certainly to grow your own foods and do organic gardening. The next best thing would be to become acquainted with the products on the label. Learn what they are and decide if you want to buy that product or not.

Write down the name of the chemicals then spend time at the library reading books on chemicals and additives.

An example of a chemical additive is Aspartame, the chemical name for NutraSweet. In their book Prescription for Nutritional Healing, J F. Balch, M.D. and Phyllis A. Balch, C.N.C., address the issue of chemical poisoning. NutraSweet "consists of three components: phenylalanine, aspartic acid, and

methanol. Because NutraSweet contains methanol, a human specific and highly toxic poison, its safety should be examined."

There are many books available at local libraries or health food stores on the subject of chemicals and the damage they do to the human body. This is a field that changes constantly because the chemicals available on the market are changing all the time. Becoming informed about your health and individual sensitivities is a personal responsibility. A little bit of knowledge goes a long way.

2. Exercise

There are two kinds of fuel used for energy when we exercise: Carbohydrates and lipids or fats. Carbohydrates are stored in the liver and skeletal muscles. Fats are stored primarily in fatty tissue.

Running to stay fit

Since exercise facilitates the burning of fat, it is a good idea to incorporate exercise on a daily basis. There are as many different types of exercise as there are people who enjoy them.

The key to exercise lies in the fact that the more you exercise (within reason), the better you feel and the better you feel the more you want to exercise.

Exercise should be strenuous enough for an individual level of fitness. It would never be advised to run 10 miles after lying around all winter without working up to it. Always exercise with wisdom. Start at a low level then work up to a higher level.

Caution: Before beginning any kind of an exercise program, include a physical exam by a qualified physician to determine your exercise capability.

Pocket book, time element, and physical fitness are all factors that need to be taken into account as you consider an exercise program.

Not only does exercise burn up fat and tone muscles, it also is very beneficial in reducing stress. Stress will be relieved as you walk and talk with someone else. Sharing lives and exercising together creates a feeling that someone cares.

On the other hand, if you are surrounded by others all day and you want some time alone, then use a brisk walk or workout at the gym for that very thing—to meditate and to heal.

Exercise is a factor in improving self-esteem. I have watched this through the years with our own children.

It all started with my husband, who was an All-American football player, and named the "All-Around" athlete of his high school his senior year. He had the ability and determination to remain athletically involved.

After a few years of marriage he recognized that he couldn't rest on old laurels, so he took up running.

He takes an hour each day from a sedentary desk job to work out at a gym or run in the mountains near where he works.

He encourages our children to keep physically fit. He has trained for and gone on fifty and twenty five mile walks with two of our daughters. He has worked with our children and has run several 5K and 10K races with them. In a later year, he and our four older boys trained together and all five of them ran a 26.2 mile marathon together. Two years later he ran with another son.

As I see the benefits of those seeds that were planted in their youth, I watch our children grow up making better choices in their personal health habits. They continue to run, bike, hike, camp, and keep themselves in good physical shape.

Sometimes when I'm watching my family run, people will ask me, "Oh, do you run, too?" My reply is, "Yes, I run them here and I run them there".

My exercise program changes with the times, the seasons and the financial situation.

Along with physical fitness, stress relief, and self esteem, posture improves with exercise. It's normal to walk straight and tall with the head erect and shoulders back. Compare that to the tired eyes, humped shoulders, and "air of discouragement" which all too often accompanies lack of physical fitness and oxygen exchange.

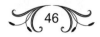

Consider the weight of gravity on our shoulders. When we slump, we carry more weight per square inch. When we walk straight and tall—straight as an arrow—it decreases the feeling of carrying the weight of the world on our shoulders.

Along with improving physical appearance, fitness and well being, relieving stress, and keeping weight under control, exercise also helps in healing. The energy that is created with exercise can be directed to a particular organ.

During exercise, use your mind to mentally gather up a ball of energy. If you have arthritis, send the ball of energy to the bones; if you have a weak heart, send it to the heart. Actually envision that organ receiving the energy and give it any healing color you wish to send to it.

Maximize the benefits of exercise by utilizing the power of your mind and the energy created during exercise.

If you have a weak heart, for instance, say to your heart, "I allow you to absorb the pink and white healing colors generated from this exercise. Take these colors and let them be directed lovingly into the DNA of every cell. I see all the valves and muscles strengthened and healthy."

This can be done with any body organ you need to work with to promote healing and strength. Use the mind's eye to see it and visually send colors and energy to it.

As has already been mentioned, exercise can facilitate the release of stress. When you are walking or running, visualize a ball of red stress flowing like a stream of water from all parts of your body into your hands. As you swing your hands, throw the ball of red stress as far as you can ahead of you.

This visualization uses both the energy of your physical body and the strong influence of your mind.

Considering the many benefits of exercise, it is important to note that exercise is not something we ever retire from. It can be a part of life as long as we live.

Exercise is for everyone!

3. Nutritional Supplements

"If I had been sick 200 years ago, I would have been better off in the hands of a medicine man of the American Indians than I would have been in those of a European physician. The Indian would have given me mental therapy, food and herb remedies. The European physician would have drained away my blood." (Quoted from "What has American Indian Medicine Given Us?" By Virgil J. Vogel, Phi Kappa Phi Journal, Spring 1991.)

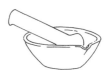

One cannot think about herbs without considering the contributions of the American Indians, the Australian Aborigine, and the highly developed cultures of the ancient Chinese in medical procedures.

Nutritional supplements

The plants all around us serve to gladden the heart, please the eye, enliven the soul and heal the body.

Even with all the groundwork that has been laid by these cultures on herbs, in modern society herbs and vitamins are constantly coming under public scrutiny. Nutritional supplements of all kinds come and go in the news media. One week they are billed as being able to heal everything; within a very short time, they are reported as being hazardous to your health.

With all this controversy, it is no wonder so many shake their heads and are dismayed as to what to do.

Let me address herbs first.

The Bible has several references to herbs. Here are a few of them:

"And God said, Behold, I have given you every herb bearing seed, which is upon the face of all the earth, and every tree, in the which is the fruit of a tree yielding seed; to you it shall be for meat." (Genesis 1:29)

"And by the river upon the bank thereof, on this side and on that side, shall grow all these for meat, whose leaf shall not fade, neither shall the fruit thereof be consumed: It shall bring forth new fruit according to his months, because their waters they issued out of the sanctuary: and the fruit thereof shall be for meat, and the leaf thereof for medicine." (Ezekiel 47:12)

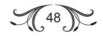

"For one believeth that he may eat all things: another, who is weak, eateth herbs. Let not him that eateth despise him that eateth not; and let not him which eateth not judge him that eateth: for God hath received him." (Romans 14:2-3)

There are those who say herbs are ineffective. Just because someone is an expert at something doesn't necessarily mean they are always right.

Good common sense is as useful today and as important as at any time in history. Many times we have to trust our own judgement.

We should not be intimidated by experts. When it comes to those things we have the most interest in, like our bodies, our families, and our personal needs, we can listen to what others say then make up our own minds.

You need to think for yourself. Study what others say and make your own judgement call. I am reminded every time I hear the story of Christopher Columbus that had he relied on the opinions of others, the world would still be flat and there would have been no discovery of the New World.

I have a client who was bitten by a spider. It's bite left four large welts on her legs and caused great concern for many well meaning friends. This lady knew deep in her heart that the best thing for her to do would be to follow an herbal program. She asked me to work with her. Every day she called to say another person scared her by saying she needed medicine. I always told her that option was certainly open to her. She continued with the herbal program and healed nicely.

She listened and made the choice that best suited her need. She did not want to be filled with a yeast infection that followed when she used antibiotics on previous occasions.

Since there are so many books available on herbs (how to gather herbs, dry them, make capsules, tinctures, herbs for decoration, herbs in cooking, etc.), I will not cover those details. Local health food stores, bookstores, and libraries will have all the information you need.

I have included a few reference books in the appendix that I have found helpful through the years.

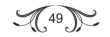

The point is that herbs ARE important. Herbs heal. Herbs have been around since God created the earth, and He gave them to us for a reason.

The same applies to vitamin and mineral supplements. We live in a day and age when our soils have become very deplete in necessary nutrients.

Our family has grown a garden for several years and we have fruit trees planted in our yard. It has been very interesting to see what has happened through the years as we eat food right out of the yard. During the months of July, August, September and early October (until the garden freezes), we test for very few vitamin or mineral supplements. However, after the Halloween holiday, there has always been a dramatic increase in our supplemental needs.

As I evaluate this, I can see the benefit of eating fresh produce right off the vine if even for a few weeks or months during the year. Each fruit or vegetable as it comes on in it's season either has a cleansing or rebuilding effect on the body. An example of this is apricots. They are the first fruit we eat in early summer (if they don't freeze first with a late spring frost). Apricots are rich in potassium and iron which are both very beneficial for the heart, blood and cells. Eating fresh apricots has a cleansing effect on the body.

Peas are typically the first vegetable to be harvested. They contain protein, iron and the B vitamins which are essential to restoring the cells, nerves and blood to optimum condition.

And so it is with each fruit or vegetable that we eat in it's season. They either cleanse or rebuild the human body.

We do need nutritional supplements. With the skills you will learn in this book, you will be able to determine your individual supplementation needs.

Herbs and vitamins will be discussed in more detail in a later chapter.

4. Sleep/rest

There is an old saying that says, "There is no rest for the wicked, and the righteous don't need it." Or, "The only place we will truly rest will be in the arms of the Lord."

Adequate sleep and rest are an important part of health.

To those of you who have babies, young children, or teenagers, your day is coming when you will be able to get adequate sleep!! (We hope!)

Some clients I work with have asked me occasionally to test them to see how much sleep they need. That is a good question because not everyone requires the same amount of sleep.

Sleep at night is vital. It allows important body functions to take place such as rest for the brain and the muscles.

Scientists have declared eight hours of sleep a night to be optimum for most people. It would be desirable if everyone needing it could sleep that long.

With Bio-Kinetic testing skills, you can now test for your individual needs, then try to work it into your schedule.

Knowing all these things doesn't make it any easier to get to sleep. There are such things as sleep apnea, insomnia, night sweats, night dreams, children, neighbors' dogs, etc., that keep you from sleeping soundly.

The best suggestions I have heard for sleeping well are these:

* If you have something to do the next day, instead of worrying about it all night, write it down on a piece of paper and mentally make a note that the next day you will get to it—if you forget something, get up and write it down, or it will play on your mind all night.

* If you have anger or negative emotions that stir you up, write a letter to whomever caused you such feelings, then get up the next morning and burn the letter. Write rapidly and don't worry about editing it or rereading it. Pour all the emotion and anger you feel onto the page. Without re-reading it the next morning, burn it. Otherwise, the anger is re-entered into your mind as you read. Just write, then burn.

* Going to sleep with a mind full of the news is going to bed with a mind full of the negative. If you feel the news bothers you, then read the scriptures or a positive-thinking book instead.

* Visualization/relaxation tapes are available. You can even ask someone with a soothing voice to record a tape for you that relaxes your mind and body. Start with the feet and let the feeling of relaxation absorb into every body part from the feet to the head.

* If you are an individual who secretes extra adrenalin during the day because of stress, a light exercise of 10-15 minutes in the evening will burn off the adrenalin and help you relax and sleep better.

Studies have been done on people who were given the chance to take a short break from work during their eight-hour shift. Those who rested worked better and more efficiently than those who pushed it hard for eight hours straight.

A quick 15-20 minute nap can be as refreshing as a whole night's sleep. You don't need to be in a bed, either. Sitting back on a chair with your feet up on a desk, reclining on a couch, or stretching out on the ground if you are an outdoor laborer are just a few of the restful positions.

5. Size and Weight

Every individual has his own metabolic rate. Learn what yours is and respect it. Some can consume chocolate and fats like they are going out of style and stay as "slender as a rail"; others claim to gain weight by simply standing in the candy bar section at the store and sniffing the sweet fumes.

One of the saddest things I have witnessed recently has been the devastating physical side effects of a popular weight-loss product that took the nation by storm. Women and men were so desperate to lose weight that some even lost their lives.

It is unrealistic to try and look like the models and artists of stage and screen who are usually undeniably trim. This makes other women start comparing themselves to what they see. It is an unreal fixation that some American men and women have about the human body.

Here are a few things I have learned about weight reduction and maintenance for those who are above optimum weight:

1. Eat less. Cut down individual serving size. Far too many of us tend to over eat rather than under eat.

2. Eat slower. Chew your food well. It is more satisfying and healthier because the food is mixed with saliva—an important step in the digestive process.

3. Limit certain fats. These include high-fat dairy products such as butter, cheese, and ice cream; deep fat fried foods like french fries, donuts, pastries, chips; fatty foods such as pie crusts, thick fatty icings, cheesecakes, cooking with shortening or fat; fatty dressings like blue cheese, ranch, mayonnaise, and sour cream.

4. Cut sugars. If it is impossible to go totally off of sugar, cut back gradually. Even that effort will make a big difference in energy levels and sugar balance.

5. Infections and hormone changes make it difficult to reduce weight; candida, or yeast, causes the body to hang onto water; a weakened pancreas contributes to an imbalance in blood sugars, which creates food cravings and eating binges; an underactive thyroid affects the metabolism; any infection or weakness in the uterus can change the hormones, causing weight retention due to hormone imbalance.

6. The pituitary gland controls the endocrine system. A whiplash or any blow to the head can upset the balance of the pituitary gland. Hormones secreted by the pituitary regulate body activities ranging from growth to reproduction. The pituitary plays an important role in the breakdown of fat, utilization of glucose, and thyroid and adrenal control, along with reproductive hormones, blood pressure, perspiration and urine output.

If you or a client test that the pituitary is out of balance, there is a way to correct it with visualization.

HOW TO RESET THE PITUITARY GLAND

Position the client in a comfortable position so he can lean back and close his eyes.

Place your right hand directly over the top of his head with your fingers resting lightly on his head. Your hand is placed so the thumb is pointing towards one ear and the remaining four fingers are towards the opposite ear.

Or, both of your hands are holding the client's feet—one hand on each foot with your thumbs resting lightly against the back of his big toes. This is the reflexology pressure point for the pituitary gland in the feet.

Instruct him to take in a deep breath and relax. Give him a second or two to respond to the suggestion.

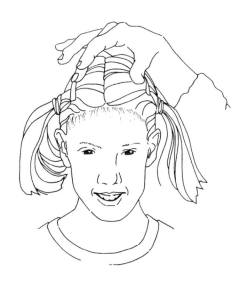

Resetting pituitary gland

Script:

> *"You are going to go on a journey down deep in your brain. If you need to, put on a miner's helmet with a light on the front.*
>
> *"As you descend into the mine, let your light flash around. Look for an organ shaped like a golf club.*
>
> *"When you find this golf club, tell me what color you see."*

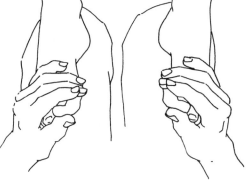

(In a previous chapter we talked about colors and their significance with regards to personal health. If he sees black or red the pituitary is definitely out of alignment.

Reflexology pressure point for the pituitary gland in the feet— thumbs lightly resting against the bottom of the big toe

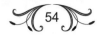

Whatever color he sees, remember the color as it will be used for comparison later.)

> *"If you had a golf club and the handle on it was bent and needed to be fixed, how would you straighten it out? Remember, it is very expensive and cannot be thrown away or replaced, but it CAN be fixed."*

(Let him describe his method for straightening something that is bent. He may put it in a vice, use his knee, step on it, use a mallet or a hammer, or bend it back with his hands. He may prefer to take it to someone else to fix—that is okay, too. If he cannot tell you how he would repair his golf club, then give him a choice of the before-mentioned methods and let him choose one.)

> *"Take the (mention the color he saw the golf club as being) and straighten it out right now.*
>
> *"When the shaft is fixed, take a bright warm torch and run it gently along the handle of the golf club you have just straightened. This reinforces and strengthens the restoration of your golf club.*
>
> *"Now what color is the golf club?"*

(Let him tell you what color he sees. The color will change to a softer hue of health.)

> *"As you breathe in that color real deep, feel the brain in the area of the pituitary filled with the glow of health.*
>
> *"Let that glow radiate inside filling the brain and cascading down through the core of your body.*
>
> *"Breathe out and say these words with me, 'healthy pituitary, healthy pituitary'.*
>
> *"When you feel like your whole body has been filled with a wonderful healing warmth, then you can take a big deep breath and open your eyes whenever you are ready."*

After experiencing this processing, some clients tell me it feels like water running down the back of their neck, others feel like a deflated basketball has been pumped up. Everyone expresses a sensation of having the brain feel lighter or cleaner.

Emotions and Weight

Along with physical balance, emotions play a big part in weight retention. Here are a few of the emotions I have run across.

- "I have things in my life YOU cannot control. I can control my body and what I eat."

- Physical abuse sets the stage for another person to "pad the body so it will not hurt so bad when I am hit."

- Early deprivation of food gave another person the feeling of, "Now I have all the food I want. I will never be hungry again."

- Using food or treats as a reward for children will instill in them as adults the idea that food (and plenty of it) is rewarding .

- Sex abuse triggered the response in another person that "I will get so big that no one will want me like that again."

If any of these circumstances apply, a good counselor is important to help bring out truths about food and body weight and dispel misconceptions.

Mental Perceptions and Weight

- The mind plays a big part in physical well-being. Use visualization to see yourself as you would like to be. Hang up a picture of how you used to look and how you would like to look again. Whatever target you aim for, you are likely to hit.

- Use phrases other than "lose weight." Think of the comparison between "losing weight" and "losing a wallet with $1000 in it." What is your natural instinct? GET IT BACK! A better choice of words could be "ideal weight" or "weight reduction" instead of "losing it."

- If you are one who likes reminders, go around the house and put up signs. "You can do it," or "Make it a pound this week," etc. Put the

signs on mirrors, cupboards or refrigerator doors. Change the signs as often as you need to. Work at it!

- Make a list of your positive strengths. Ask those who would be kind to you what they like about you. It helps to hear an honest compliment. The body will respond and want to be what others say you are and can become.

- You need a good reason to look nice, or someone you want to look nice for. A husband, a boyfriend, a class reunion, a summer bikini, or wedding reception line are good enough reasons. Consider, also, your health, energy or self esteem and how they will benefit from reaching and maintaining optimum weight.

Think of yourself as a marathon runner and not a sprinter in dealing with excess weight. My husband has to pace himself in a marathon run or he will run out of steam before reaching his goal. Decide right now that you would rather reach an ideal weight slowly and form good habits to keep if off, than to get over anxious and then become discouraged. Aesop's fable of the tortoise and the hare is a good example. Those who work at weight reduction slow and systematically, without giving up, become the winners.

Weight maintenance programs exist. With Bio-Kinetic testing skills you will be able to find which one is best for you. Herbs can be customized for a weight-maintenance program once you learn how to test for them.

In the section at the end of the book called FREQUENTLY ASKED QUESTIONS (FAQs) you will find a list of herbs you can test for as you begin an individual weight-maintenance program and suggestions on how to follow this list.

CHILDREN LEARN WHAT THEY LIVE

by Dorothy Law Nolte

If children live with criticism, they learn to condemn.
If children live with hostility, they learn to fight.
If children live with ridicule, they learn to be shy.
If children live with shame, they learn to feel guilty.
If children live with tolerance, they learn to be patient.
If children live with encouragement, they learn confidence.
If children live with praise, they learn to appreciate.
If children live with fairness, ,they learn justice.
If children live with security, they learn to have faith.
If children live with approval, they learn to like themselves.
If children live with acceptance and friendship,
they learn to find love in the world.

EMOTIONAL

Health is not just absence of disease. More than ever health is becoming the ability to find peace in a troubled world.

Medical doctors and psychologists alike have tried to understand why one person can be exposed to a disease organism and they get sick, while another exposed to the same organism can resist it.

So what is health? The World Health Organization (WHO) describes health as a "state of well-being, not just the absence of disease."

Social interaction has a lot to do with emotional health. A study done several years ago in a little town in Pennsylvania emphasized this point.

The people there had half the cardiovascular (heart) disease of the rest of the nation.

Curious public health teams descended upon this town thinking they would find citizens exercising, eating their salads, and living lives exemplary as to what is expected by all medically aware groups for good health and long lives.

What they found was a surprise. It was a small Italian-American community. The people were basically overweight with the same high blood pressure as the rest of us. They were not rigorously exercising, and their diet was the same as ours.

Love Makes a Difference

What made the difference? Upon closer evaluation, it was determined that these folks lived in a close-knit community where they had strong family structures and ties. There were extended family members who could love and support the children as they grew up; that task was not left entirely up to a mother and father. There was someone to share sorrow and joy who really cared.

What they had was a feeling of belonging, of being loved. This seems to be a bigger element in some ways than all the physical advice being handed out. (Taken from the article, "Good Health: More Than Absence of Disease",

Deseret News, LDS Church News, as quoted by N. Lee Smith, M.D., November 13, 1993)

There has been significant research done on the affect of social support along with the positive power of love, hugs, smiles, words of encouragement and happy marriages on longevity and personal health.

Positive Attitude

Along with this, health is dependent upon your feeling like you are a part of your environment, that you are important and that you make a difference by being in the world.

The native American Indians taught and passed on to their posterity the importance of being at peace with and respecting the environment. Our environment today consists of many of the same elements they enjoyed such as mountains, trees, rivers, oceans, and animals. It just includes something they did not have—more crowds and closer living conditions.

With the stress of congested freeways and suburbs, it is more important than ever to find peace in, and compatibility with, this new environment. It is still possible. Peace is not found in just the outward living places. It is found within an individual.

Stress-resilient people are able to come through a difficult situation and make the best or look for the best in it, using it as a learning experience instead of a battering ram.

Emotionally healthy people will find love and respect for their fellow man instead of looking for and finding only the ugly and bad. Personal self-esteem is enhanced as we look for the good qualities in others. Both the good and the bad are out there, it depends on where you look.

Emotional health also has much to do with how you view yourself. Do you love and respect yourself for who you are and your personal talents and abilities, or are you one who is always comparing yourself to another and feeling quite cheated and inadequate?

Emotional health really translates into one of the biggest words of our vocabulary: LOVE; Love of self, God, and fellow man.

Elizabeth Kubler-Ross, author of On Death and Dying, made this statement for "Parade Magazine," in an articled entitled, "To Be Whole Again," page 10, August 11, 1991:

> "If we could raise one generation of children
> with unconditional love, there would be no Hitlers."

This is a very profound statement. Think of how different this world would be if just one generation of children were to be raised in moral purity, health, and happiness.

Child Abuse

The sad fact remains that too many children are being abused, neglected, emotionally shattered, and exposed to harsh things that force them into an adult world they are ill prepared to cope with. Children should be allowed to be children. Nothing pains humanity more than the pain of little children.

When I worked as a nurse in a community hospital, I spent some time in the pediatrics ward. What I witnessed there would many times drive me from the room in tears. I saw children whose battered and beaten bodies lie in pain and agony while parents claimed they had fallen down stairs. One sweet little girl I saw had cigarette burns all over her body. She had been used as an ash tray.

Jesus Christ made a statement to those who would do this to little children:

> *"But whoso shall offend one of these little ones which believe in me,*
> *it were better for him that a millstone were hanged about his neck,*
> *and that he were drowned in the depth of the sea.*

> *"Woe unto the world because of offences! For it must needs be that*
> *offences come; but woe to that man by whom the offence cometh!"*
> *(Matthew 18:5-7)*

The saddest commentary on this is what these innocent ones grow up to be. We all pay a high price as they enter society.

From the counseling and work I have done with emotional healing, it is my observation that when a child is sexually or physically abused, their maturity or emotional growth is stunted at that age. The body continues to grow and

mature but their ability to deal with adult issues does not progress at the same rate.

For instance, if a girl is sexually abused at age three, she will grow up into a physically attractive woman but will see the world through the eyes of a three-year-old. How many three-year-olds are able to drive a car, hold down a job, or even survive in high school?

What I see happening to these children as they face the conflict between what society expects from someone their age and what they are really capable of doing is rebellion, drug abuse, sexual promiscuity, running away from home, anger, abuse against others, alcoholism, school truancies, and any number of unacceptable social behaviors.

So, what can be done about this?

The first step to overcoming abuse is to acknowledge that it actually happened.

Here are some indications physical, sexual, or emotional abuse MAY have occurred:

- Uncontrolled angers. The abused victim expresses what feels like a "caged tiger inside trying to burst free but never able to." Of course, the child was angry when he was violated but was never able to express it. Feelings that went unexpressed at the time come out later in the form of angers or rage.

- Unusual defiance. They will stand strong against anything that feels like someone is trying to control them, even when a suggestion is made in love. Sex abuse is a control issue and defying anyone who tries to enforce a simple rule later in life becomes one way of subconsciously speaking out against the forced control that took place during abuse.

- High divorce rate or dissatisfaction with marriage. A memory of something they did not want surfaces every time a spouse approaches with sexual intent, no matter how loving. Any sexual partner subconsciously embodies the abuser.

- Sexual promiscuity. Remember that the grown up child or person you see is still a small child acting out what was taught to him at an early age.

- Emotional outbursts. They will burst out in tears or be very fearful of situations. This has a lot to do with individual treatment during abuse. A child who is choked, shaken, or threatened into silence will release all those emotions later at the slightest "trigger" or stimulus.

- Painful intercourse, menstrual cramps, and/or childbirth. All of these recreate a painful memory.

- Distrust of either sex. Underlying criticisms of or strong dislike or distrust of men (or women if the perpetrator was female).

- Antidepressants, drugs or substance abuse of any kind that dull the memory become a part of their life. This becomes a way of trying to dull a persistent memory. Using mind and nerve altering substances to forget abuse is like trying to bury an elephant in the backyard.

- Fierce competition. This is their way of trying to prove how strong they are. The message here is, "I will get so strong that no one will ever do that to me again!"

- Homosexuality or bisexual tendencies. The first experience with sex is imprinted on the mind of the child. If the perpetrator was a man abusing a boy or a female abusing a girl, homosexual tendencies may develop. We always remember the first person who introduced us to sexual pleasures.

- Unusually passive or subdued. Brutal abuse can take away the spontaneity, self-esteem and joy of living that children naturally come with.

- Sexual fantasies. When children are abused, they mentally remove themselves from the situation in an attempt to be able to survive the trauma. This can set the pattern for later sexual relations where their mind automatically sets the stage to escape into a fantasy or pretend world.

- Lies. There have been children who have lied and made up stories about sexual abuse. It is usually to get attention or draw attention away from a bigger issue in their life. A wise parent will know their

child well enough to notice "stories" that are not true. A family I know have a grown and married daughter who accused her father of sexually abusing her. It was very traumatic for the family. It was discovered later that she had been abused, but by someone other than her father.

- Stealing and/or hiding things. It is very frustrating for a parent who can provide something for their child, to have them steal it from a store. A victim of abuse had a childhood stolen from them and this is their way of trying to steal it back. They will also hide things in their room or verbally hide emotions and feelings.

- Bad dreams, restless at night, can't sleep. The subconscious mind draws up images and memories when the conscious mind is in a resting state. This occurs mostly at night. With sex abuse, the perpetrator usually uses darkness to cover his deeds. Thus, nighttime, subconsciously, becomes a dreaded memory for the victims. One of my clients is an older woman who was sexually abused by a step father until she was old enough to begin her menstrual cycle. She has used the strongest sleeping medications and relaxants available through prescription in an attempt to sleep. They don't work because her subconscious nighttime memory is stronger than any medication.

The next step is to seek help from a good counselor who would never exercise control or put suggestions in the minds of the innocent, but would serve, instead, as a gentle mediator who allows the truth to surface on it's own.

There are estimates that at least fifty percent of this earth's children are sexually abused before they grow to adulthood. The numbers are staggering. Think of the adults out there who look and act normal but deep inside are hurting. They need to know how others have coped.

Carlfred Broderick, a noted counselor with experiences in church responsibilities and family counseling said,

> *"God actively intervenes in some destructive lineages, assigning a valiant spirit to break the chain of destructiveness in such families. Although these children may suffer innocently as victims of violence, neglect, and exploitation, through the grace of God some find the strength to 'metabolize' the poison within themselves, refusing to pass it on to future generation. Before them were generations of destructive pain; after them the line flows clear and*

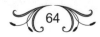

pure. Their children and their children's children will call them blessed.

In suffering innocently that others might not suffer, such persons, in some degree, become as 'saviors on mount Zion' by helping to bring salvation to a lineage.

In a former era, the Lord sent a flood to destroy unworthy lineages. In this generation, it is my faith that he has sent numerous choice individuals to help purify them."

Recognize that healing CAN and does take place.

Healing sessions with my clients who have experienced abuse have pointed out that positive personality traits are also brought out.

Some of these are:
- Compassion for others who are suffering. Personal experience helps them relate to the feelings of others have who have been traumatized in some way.

- The gift of discernment. This is an awareness of who or what is safe or unsafe to be around.

- A desire to protect little children. The injured child in them wants to make life safe for other little children.

- Wisdom beyond their years. They have an incredible understanding of and acceptance of life.

- A sure knowledge of Jesus Christ. In every case, when a child is abused, Jesus Christ is there. He holds, nurtures and loves the little spirit while the abuse is going on.

- Strong gifts or talents are developed. A special friend of mine had gone through terrible sexual and emotional abuse as a child at the hands of his parents. As he grew up he lost his sight as a direct result of the abuse. After a turbulent early adulthood, he found the martial arts. He also found a wonderful lady who loved and understood his pain, for her path had been very similar. He not only knew martial defense but taught it. No one could defeat him.

As a result of his vision impairment he developed the ability to "see" light movements, somewhat like a bat senses with it's radar. He could tell who entered the room by the "color" or sense of the individual. One day I asked, "What color am I?" He responded, "You are like a refined gold." I raised my hands to look at my rings to determine if I could see what color gold he was referring to. He said, "Not that color of gold." He had "seen" my movement.

Not only did he heal from his trauma, he became productive and reached into the life of so many others with his strength and love.

If a child says he has been abused—BELIEVE HIM!!

ODE TO THE CHILD ABUSER

by Tisha Mecham
October 1992

Why did you betray me?
I did nothing to hurt you.
Why did you fill my childhood years
With things only adults should do?
You have turned my joy to sorrow;
Left my body racked with pain.
Deep within my heart I wonder
"Will my life ever be the same?"
What you did to me was naughty.
What you did was not so nice!
Anyone who defiles a child
Will one day pay the price.
You will meet our Great Creator
To account for dastardly deeds
Where all thoughts of stolen childhood
Bring a villain to his knees.
I stand in purest innocence!
I'm a child who's done nothing wrong.
I know God in His mercy
Will reach down and keep me strong.
I shall rise with Him in glory
As the child I used to be
Learns to love and trust again.
I WILL NOT let you destroy me!!

Parenting

Knowing that abuse does and will exist in the world, it becomes the responsibility of every adult to be aware of better ways to teach, warn and raise our children.

Don't you wish when babies were born they would come with their own instruction manual tucked away somewhere? Now there's an idea! Since that can't be done, the next best thing is to make parenting a study by attending classes or reading about good parenting skills. Church organizations, public groups and PTA's offer classes to teach parents how to be parents. None of us were ever parents before at this particular time of our lives or under these particular circumstances, so it helps to learn from others who have already walked that path.

Circumstances change with age, birth of a child, becoming a grandparent; and, since we only have one chance to live, let's do our best.

Watching how others handle their children helps, and if you like their method, use it in your home.

Listen to the Children!

When TV or ball games become more important than the needs of a child, you are missing the golden opportunities.

I have listened many times to grown women and men go back in their memory to a childhood—not of abuse, but of uninvolved parents. Through their tears they tell their mother or dad, "Just spend some time with me!"

Attend Their Important Occasions

When a child has put forth time to practice a play at school, worked hard to develop music, sports or any other talent or skill, the least you can do is be there in loving support.

Cook Meals

There was a phrase coined in the 1960s that said, "The family that prays together, stays together." What better time to pray together than around a well-planned meal.

It gives a child security and comfort when you fulfill one of the responsibilities of parenthood to provide a good meal for your family.

When Possible, Mothers Need to be Home with Their Children

This is a day and age when many mothers have to work to help support the family. However, if a mother works to get away from home responsibility or pay for expensive homes, boats or vacation trips, then consider if those are really more important than forging the self-esteem and love of an individual who will grow into productive adulthood.

Children are only children for a few short years. All too soon they have grown and left the nest in a flurry.

Strengthen the Chakra

One of the reasons it is so important for an adult to be in the presence of her child deals with the chakra, or energy fields.

When a baby is born, his chakra are not fully developed. He draws upon the energy of loved ones around him until he is old enough to have explored the world and had experiences of his own.

In her book, *Hands of Light*, Barbara Ann Brennan points out that the crown chakra (or spiritual) of a newborn is wide open whereas the root chakra, or physical, is less developed.

During this time, while the child is growing "roots" to the earth or physical plane, he needs to feel loved, accepted, and secure. This is done when he is sheltered in the presence of a strong, constant adult chakra.

"At about age seven a protective screen is formed over the chakra openings" and this makes the child more independent, able to reason and venture out more on his own.

Another study suggests that the brain of a child accepts everything as truth until about age seven or eight, at which time he develops reasoning ability and can sort truth from error.

For example, if a dad says to his 3 year old, "Button that shirt. You are so slow." The child says to himself, "I'm slow". However, at age 7—8 when dad says, "Button that shirt. You are so slow." The child is now able to use his reasoning ability with, "Dad must be in a hurry".

Keep a Level Head and Sense of Humor

Nothing defrays a tough situation faster than seeing the humor in it. Of course, there are times when laughing is just not appropriate, but with most of life's day to day happenings, look on the bright side. So the car runs out of gas in the middle of a freeway. When this happened, I had the pleasure of pushing it to the next exit (slightly downhill) while my 15 year old—not yet old enough to drive—daughter sat behind the wheel and "drove" to the off ramp. I reminded her that when she did get to drive, this was as fast as she would be allowed to travel.

The Emotional/Physical Health

Emotional illness can often cause physical illness, whether real or imagined.

Physical and emotional health are closely related.

I have worked with people who are absolutely well physically but cannot get out of bed because of emotional stress.

Ask yourself these questions:

"Do I like to have others wait on me?"

"Does illness relieve decision making?"

"Do I get more attention and help when I am sick?"

It is a fact that the sickest person is the one who controls a household or a situation.

One case I encountered of emotional/physical illness dealt with a woman whose parents had separated when she was very young. Her mother had to go to work and the only time she could stay home with her daughter was during times of childhood illness. Hence, a subconscious desire developed in the daughter to be ill; for illness got her what she REALLY wanted.

I am not saying we should neglect our children when they are sick. However, it would be wise to not let illness or being home in bed something that becomes comfortable.

Talk to your child about the illness. Validate his feelings and allow him to express how he feels. A possible dialogue could be, "No one likes to be sick."

"Let's see what we can do to help you feel well again."

"Does your tummy hurt? I'm so sorry. I don't like it when I hurt, either. I like being healthy. It's more fun, isn't it?"

Children are good at "faking" illness if there is an uncomfortable situation at school or if they are not prepared for a test.

We had a fast rule at our home: "If you are too sick to go to school, you are too sick to go any place else." If friends came around after school, a sick child could not play because that was part of "being sick."

Earlier training lays the foundation for adult actions and behaviors. If illness becomes an excuse early in life, it becomes a way to skirt issues and not face things directly as the child matures. Many hours are lost by the work force because of illness. This is a big loss to any business.

It would be a financial boon to our country if everyone learned the skills of Bio-Kinetic testing and stayed on the job.

In 1997 I spent three hours an afternoon every other week testing employees of a large corporation. Their manager allowed them a 20 minute break, they would come into an empty room and be tested, then return to work.

One of the employees sent a sign-up list around so when I got there it was already scheduled. The health of those individuals improved dramatically.

Their complaints of being too tired to go to work, or individual aches and pains began to fade. There were some who overcame irritability with other employees.

What a wonderful price to pay for better health and relations in a work environment. Learning the skills of Bio-Kinetics will enable you to be a better employee or employer.

HEALTH IS WEALTH!!

POINTS TO PONDER

If you don't like the weather, wait 10 minutes and it will change

The best things in life aren't things

Those who live with the most toys still die

If you never felt rain you would never see the rainbow

The two ways to be rich are: Make more money or desire less things

True beauty is internal —looks mean nothing.

Consider Noah: He worked 100 years to build his ship then only floated it once.

Pray to know your personal truth—then live it

Age is relative—once you're over the hill you pick up speed

Hook your wagon to a star

Hug life and take time to smell the roses

Before ye seek for riches, seek ye first the kingdom of God and all things shall be added unto you

Draw hearts and smiles on everything

No one ever saw the sun by looking down

The best way to swallow an elephant is a bite at a time

MENTAL

One time a youth said to Socrates, "Master, how can I get knowledge?"

Socrates said, "Do you want to get knowledge?"

"Yes, tell me how to get it."

Socrates said, "Come with me."

He took him by the hand, and led him out of the building.

The boy thought to himself, "Where could we be going to get knowledge outside of the building?"

When they came to a stream, the boy said, "Where are we going to get knowledge out here?"

Socrates said nothing. Still holding the youth's hand, they walked into the water up to his waist. Then Socrates held the one hand and put his other hand on the boy's head. And the boy said, "Surely he is going to give me a blessing and show me how to get knowledge."

He gave him a blessing all right! He shoved the boy's head under the water, and held him there. The boy squirmed and he kicked and tried to get his head up. Socrates was strong, and he held him there.

Just as the boy was ready to pass out, Socrates pulled him up. Socrates said, "When you want knowledge as badly as you wanted air just now, you'll get knowledge."

This story has been passed down through time, and has been repeated on many different occasions, both over pulpits and in classrooms. The moral of the story is well taken.

There are four aspects of mental health I would like to address:
1) knowledge 2) positive thinking 3) goal setting 4) meditation

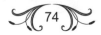

Knowledge

1. Not very many of us have to struggle like the poor youth at the hands of
    Socrates to gain knowledge. Education is currently available to all who
    desire it. We have moved into a highly educated society compared to
    earlier centuries where children were required to work on family farms
    or in factories instead of getting an education. Laws today require that
    children attend school.

The mental area of health has a lot to do with basic book work, such as grades,
homework and studies. This is where we obtain most knowledge. However, it
doesn't stop there.

An education is available in a high school or college, and is also available in an
office, the home, or a factory. It is the willingness to learn and a desire to
acquire knowledge and advance that gives one an education.

Knowledge is potential power. Knowledge becomes power when wisdom is
applied. There are two aspects to knowledge: one is knowledge and the other
is wisdom. Knowledge is knowing how a car works; wisdom is putting it into
gear and driving it away. Wisdom is the application of knowledge.

King Solomon in the Bible was well-known for his wisdom. It is a high
compliment to say someone has "the wisdom of Solomon."

Solomon became king after his father, King David, died. He considered
himself but a youth and asked God to help him with the mantle of kingship
that he judge the people wisely.

God was pleased with him and said,

> *"Because thou has . . . not asked for thyself long life; neither hast
> asked riches for thyself, nor hast asked the life of thine enemies; but
> hast asked for thyself understanding to discern judgement; behold,
> I have done according to thy words: Lo, I have given thee a wise
> and an understanding heart . . . (1 Kings 3:11 -12)*

> *"And Solomon's wisdom excelled the wisdom of all the children of
> the east country, and all the wisdom of Egypt. For he was wiser
> than all men . . . and his fame was in all nations round about.*

"He spake three thousand proverbs: and his songs were a thousand and five.

"And there came of all people to hear the wisdom of Solomon, from all kings of the earth, which had heard of his wisdom." (1 Kings 4:29- 34.)

He became most famous for his judgement between two women who claimed to be the mother of a living child. Each woman said a child who had died earlier was the child of the other.

As Solomon listened to the women, he calmly commanded that the living child be brought in. He then asked for a sword and said he would cut the child in two and give half to each woman.

One woman said,

"O my lord, give her the living child, and in no wise slay it. But the other said, Let it be neither mine nor thine, but divide it." (1 Kings 3:16-27)

The king was quite aware that a true mother would rather give a child away than see it slain. His wisdom in this decision was legendary.

It is the desire of every parent on earth that their children gain knowledge and wisdom.

There is a difference between simply knowing what is right and wrong and having the wisdom to DO what is right.

Positive Thinking

2.   There are many who are skilled in writing and speaking about positive thinking. Best known for this is Dr. Norman Vincent Peale. He has been a motivating force for the better in the lives of many. His books are very uplifting and worth reading. If you are a negative thinker, you CAN change that trend.

Positive thinking has a big impact on personal health. You cannot be healthy and constantly thinking of ailments and sickness.

Thinking positive is like shaving, no matter how good a job you do of it today, it still needs to be done tomorrow.

Positive thinkers are optimists. When I meet a really great individual who seems so modest and yet strong in his field, it gives me faith in my own possibilities.

Negative thinking is a bad habit, but habits can be broken. Bad habits are almost like a comfortable bed, easy to get in to but hard to get out of.

On the other hand, positive thinking is a wonderful sensation you acquire when you are too busy to be miserable.

Goal Setting

3. Setting goals is a good practice to follow. Some people set daily goals, some use yearly achievements, and others follow their stars into the future. However you set a goal, it is important to evaluate it occasionally and see how you are progressing.

As a family, we sit down together the first Monday of every new year and write goals for the coming year. These goals are typed and displayed in a prominent place in our front room. Every visitor or interested person who wants to can read those goals. This is a stimulus to accomplish at least one of the goals for so many people see it and hold us to our commitments.

From the poem *Invictus* came these stirring words:

> In the fell clutch of circumstances, I have not
> Winced or cried aloud.
> Under the bludgeoning of chance, my head is
> Bloody but unbowed.
> It matters not how straight the gate, how charged
> With punishment the scroll.
> I am the Master of my Fate, I am the
> Captain of my soul.

If you don't set goals and make life happen, then you become a victim of life itself and will be moved whichever direction it desires to move you.

There is a much-quoted saying, "What you are today is God's gift to you, but that which you become is your gift to God." (Anon.) To become something, set a goal and work for it.

Meditation

4.   Meditation is sitting quietly, tuning out distractions, then conversing with yourself or a Higher Being.

There are various forms of meditation. Each person should find the one that best suits his needs. Meditation can be done by sitting in a quiet room breathing deeply and relaxing or it can be accomplished during an exercise routine.

Our minds become so full of distractions and negative thoughts that we need to take time to "clear the air", so to speak.

Meditation can be done with tapes or prerecorded scripts. It helps to have someone else's voice walk us through a session.

Prayer is a form of meditation. It is getting in contact with a Higher Being and feeling the flow of energy as we ask questions and get answers.

To use prayer as a form of meditation, the number one rule is: The prayer needs to last longer than thirty seconds.

Recently I heard of a form of meditation. It spoke of a school in China where the children sit and face the east. In this position they make sweeping motions with their hands on each side of the head.

When asked what they were doing, the schoolmaster said they were using the prevailing breeze and sweeping away the negative from their brains. They would meditate about removing the impure and replacing it with clean and pure thoughts. This was facilitated by the gentle, clear breeze blowing in off the ocean.

In this world where we are surrounded by so many people and pressures, it is important to take time for ourselves. One of the best things we can do is to spend time with ourselves in thought, introspection, and strengthening positive images.

HEAVEN'S VIEW

By
Donna Miesbach

Some say that God's invisible.
I have another view.
I see Him every passing day –
He smiles at me through you!

He comforts me when I am sad
Through every loving word you say,
And when my cares seem heaviest,
Your presence drives them all away.

The tender touch of your dear hand
Is but His angel-kiss,
And every thoughtful thing you do
Reflects sweet heaven's bliss.

No need to wait for heaven
To get a better view
When I can see His loving glance
Each time I look at you!

— *Unity Magazine*
July 1984

SPIRITUAL

Lucky is the man, woman, or child who has faith in someone more loving, kind, and wise than himself.

There was a story told of an old Indian chief whose son was raised to have faith in the Great Spirit. The son went away to college and upon returning had a different attitude about this teaching. He now believed that one had to see something to believe in its reality.

After trying in vain to rekindle some faith in his son, the father and son went to spend time alone in the mountains.

Early the next morning the son came running to his father and said, "There was a bear in camp last night!"

"Oh," questioned the father "How do you know? I don't see a bear."

"Well, look, there are tracks all over. It's evident that a bear has been around," the eager son responded.

"And so it is with the Great Spirit," said his wise father, "I don't see him but as I look around this world, I see His tracks everywhere. I see it in the sunrise, the eagle, and the tender leaf of every tree."

There are many books that are more eloquent than I in describing the way to find God.

God is the creator of all. He is the giver and taker of life. Everything we do is done under His direction. To be a healer, you need to recognize and respect eternal energies.

Healing is a special gift. It is a call from God to be His hands on earth.

HEALER

Past the seeker as he prayed,
Came the crippled and the beggar
and the beaten.
And seeing them, the holy one went
down into deep prayer and cried:
"Great One, how is it that a
Loving Creator can see such things
and yet do nothing about them?"
And out of the long silence, God said,
I did do something, I made you."
— *(Anonymous)*

Even if you have no wish to enter the healing experience, or work on others, personal health is greatly enhanced by a faith in God.

In the Holy Bible, the book of Isaiah points this out:

"But they that wait upon the Lord shall renew their strength; they shall mount up with wings as eagles; they shall run, and not be weary; and they shall walk, and not faint." (Isaiah 40:31)

A belief in God is synonymous with the early fiber of the American Nation. The pilgrims and Puritans came here mainly seeking religious freedom.

When prayers and God's name were removed from our public schools and meeting places, we began a step in the direction of disrespect and an increase in crime and violence.

The law of opposites declares how hard it is to be on both ends of the spectrum. For example, you cannot be sad and yet happy at the same time; it is impossible to be rich and poor at the same time; you cannot travel north and south at the same time; and neither is it possible to worship God and live in wickedness at the same time.

To create an atmosphere of faith and love, it must be done in God's name. Ignore God, you ignore all His goodness. He never leaves us alone, but He waits patiently for us to find Him.

To get a feel for the great loving goodness of Jesus Christ and God the Father, I would recommend reading the book *Return From Tomorrow* by George G. Ritchie. He tells of meeting Christ after suffering "death" through an illness. As Mr. Ritchie describes his experience, the one thing that is most prominent is the great and eternal love of Christ.

Having experienced that love, Mr. Ritchie returned with a determination to emulate that love to others and to help his fellow-man.

A belief in God and a belief that life goes on even after death has a positive effect on how daily affairs are carried out. It would ease many of our social ills if more of us lived each day as if we were about to meet our Creator tomorrow.

From a book of quotations that I have collected through the years, I gathered these sayings from unknown sources:

> Abraham Lincoln said, "We trust, Sir, that God is on our side. It is more important to know that we are on God's side."

> Augustine: "I searched the world over for God and found Him in my heart."

> Nathaniel Hawthorn: "Whoever thinks long enough in terms of Christ, acts long enough in terms of Christ, lives long enough in terms of Christ, will in the end become like Christ."

The supreme example of healing is my Mentor and Friend, Jesus Christ. With hands outstretched He blessed all who came to Him seeking help.

> "Is any sick among you? Let him call for the elders of the church; and let them pray over him, anointing him with oil in the name of the Lord:

> And the prayer of faith shall save the sick, and the Lord shall raise him up; and if he have committed sins, they shall be forgiven him." (James 5:14—15)

The master healer works through us. We are but the hands of Christ on earth. Always give healing credit where credit is due.

When I work on clients who have been diagnosed with terminal illnesses, I say to them, "Where God is concerned, what does man know anyway?" We do all we can by using vitamins and herbs and dietary changes knowing full well the ultimate healing is under God's direction. With the healing arts you will begin to feel an upsurge of understanding and teaching take place. A willing heart combined with skills and a desire to help another who is sick or downtrodden, automatically invites divine intervention.

Anytime you are working on one of God's children, He will not leave you to work alone.

Any desire that matches the heart, goes up in a prayer.

A spiritual awareness is as vital to healing as a space ship is to an astronaut.

When dealing with your own or another's health issues, work with all four areas of health to promote total healing.

> *"Give a man an incurable disease, let him take care of it, and he will live a long time."*
>
> — *Heber C. Kimball*

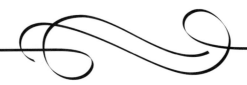

HEALTH RAP

by Tisha Mecham

Meshach, Shadrach, and Abednego
Were friends of Daniel a long time ago.
King Nebuchadnezzar—he was the one—he said
"Come to my palace, boys, and have some fun!!
Eat all this food. Drink all this drink!!"
But Daniel said, "Hey man, I can't think!
My body's not made for all this JUNK,
I wanna grow up and be a 'big hunk'.
Bring on the veggies, the fruit and the seeds.
Cut out the dead foods, if you please."
So these four boys, they did their thing
And grew ten times smarter than the dudes of the king.
Smarter and stronger you're gonna be.
Just treat you body like sacred pro-per-ty.
Oh, yeah

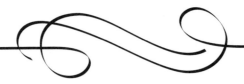

CHAPTER 6

Understanding Your Body

To be able to use the skills of Bio-Kinetic testing, be aware that you will be able to test only as far as personal knowledge will allow. As with anything, the basic law is "the more you understand, the better you are".

This does not imply that only the learned can do the testing. My objective is to reach everyone, for these skills belong to ALL who seek.

This is not going to be a detailed medical course. As you will see, it is a brief description of the location and function of body parts.

There are many books written on nearly every subject possible about the human body. Time and space do not allow me to give you the depth of knowledge that some of you may want to acquire. I suggest visiting your library or attending a local college if you want more information.

The whole objective of this material is to stimulate an interest in personal health and provide some working knowledge of your body. If I err in my information, it is not done intentionally. I am open to suggestions or information, for are we not all students of life?

There are many things that are yet to be understood by medical science. Much has been, and much more will continue to be brought to light concerning the working of the most perfect creation—the human body.

The illustrations in this manual will be sufficient to give you a basic understanding of the anatomy to begin testing. Studying the pictures will fix

an image in your mind of that body part, how it looks, and where it is located. It is important to have at least an idea of the specific body part and it's basic function in order to work with Bio-Kinetic skills.

THE SKELETAL SYSTEM

The bones give the body shape. Some bones serve to protect delicate organs. Some bones are held together with ligaments and form joints so we can move freely; other bones have slight or no movement. The back bones, or spine, protect the spinal chord, which carries nerve impulses back and forth from the brain to the body.

If the bones of the back are out of alignment, you can expect to have a variety of ailments. Nerves radiate off the spinal column and carry electrical impulses to corresponding organs of the body.

Bones have growth plates that cause children to complain of leg aches during periods of growth. The most obvious are those just below the knee. The lower leg bones grow down from these growth plates.

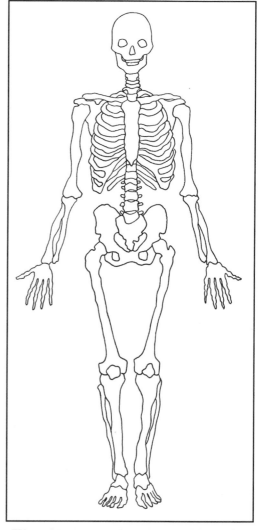

The Human Skeletal System

MUSCLES

Muscle mass makes up 40-50 percent of body weight. Muscles come in three types: voluntary, involuntary and smooth. Voluntary muscles can be controlled. These muscles are attached to bones and allow us to walk across a room, throw a ball, give a hug, or any motion that requires action and conscious thought. Involuntary muscles function without even thinking about it. An example of this is the heart muscle. Smooth muscles are in the stomach, blood vessels, intestines, and other hollow internal structures (these are also considered involuntary).

Muscles are important for the movement necessary in physical activities, moving substances in the body, helping us keep any given position like sitting or standing, and regulation of heat and body temperature.

Muscles can be pulled or sprained, which causes pain.

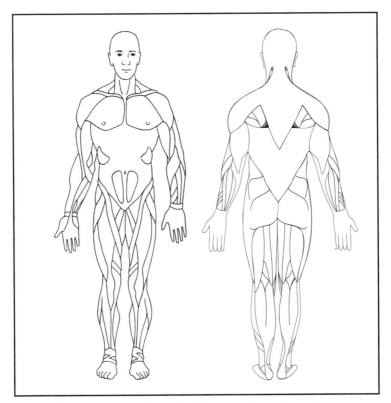

Front and Back Muscular System

BRAIN

The brain is one of the largest organs of the body. It is divided into four sections: the cerebrum, the cerebellum, the brain stem, and the diencephalon or thalamus/hypothalamus area. It is also divided into the left and right hemispheres.

The brain controls all the body's voluntary and involuntary activities. It is the center of thought, memory, emotion, and language.

The cerebrum is where most conscious and intelligent activities are created; the brain stem controls functions such as breathing and digestion; the cerebellum controls posture and coordinates body movements; diencephalon is deep inside the brain where the thalamus and hypothalamus are contained. These are important for sensory impulse transmission, homeostasis, certain emotions such as anger, pleasure, pain, etc., and the hunger and thirst control.

(Illustration # 18)

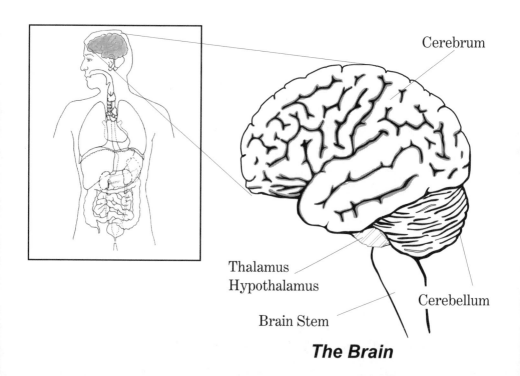

The Brain

EYES

The eyes are vital to sight. The eyes consist of the eyeballs, eyelids, eyebrows, and tear ducts. Optic nerves conduct images from the retina to the brain where images are produced. The iris constricts and expands to control light exposure.

Nearsightedness is when the light rays or images focus short of the retina. This restricts vision to near or close-up range. Farsightedness is when light rays focus beyond the normal distance of the retina. Farsighted persons can see a bee on a leaf a mile away, so to speak, but can't read a book at 12 inches. Both of these conditions require corrective reading lenses.

As you know, iridology is the science of reading the body's energy through the eyes. There are nerve endings from all parts of the body that end in the eyes. Bio-Kinetic testing uses this same energy. However, with Bio-Kinetics it is possible to pinpoint exact details of illness and supplements to help the body heal.

Emotions and feelings are usually easy to see in the eyes. When you become in tune to an individual you can tell immediately by looking in his eyes whether he is happy, sad or angry. The eyes are the window of the soul because they reflect the true inner personality.

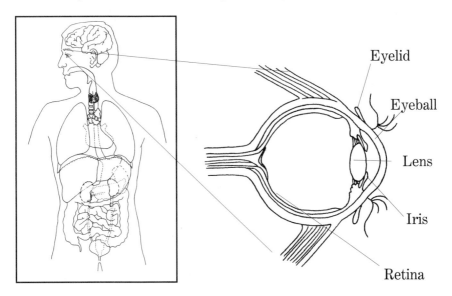

The Eye

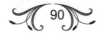

EARS

The ears allow us to hear and maintain equilibrium or balance. The outer ear is the visible appendage on the head and the ear canal. The middle ear is inside the head and contains the eustachian tube, which balances pressure on both sides of the eardrum, and three tiny bones called the malleus, incus, and stapes. These convey sound vibrations to the inner ear.

The inner ear contains the semicircular canals and cochlea. The fluid and tiny hairs in the semicircular canals help maintain balance.

Allergies and infections in the semicircular canals cause dizziness and/or nausea as they interfere with the cilia and fluid function.

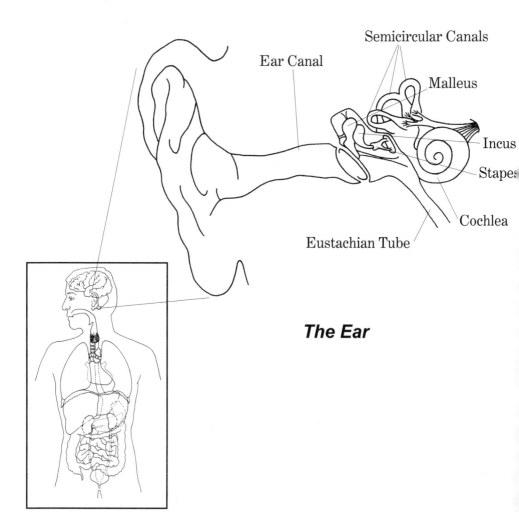

The Ear

NOSE/THROAT

Sinus cavities are situated above and below the eyes. These are bony cavities that assist in breathing. Infection or allergy in the sinuses builds up painful mucous and pressure.

The nasal cavity warms and moistens the air, and the tiny hairs protect against foreign bodies.

The tongue assists with swallowing and detecting taste differentiation in bitter, sour, salty, and sweet.

Saliva secreted from the salivary glands lubricates food and begins the chemical breakdown in the digestive process. Food should be chewed slowly and mixed well with saliva.

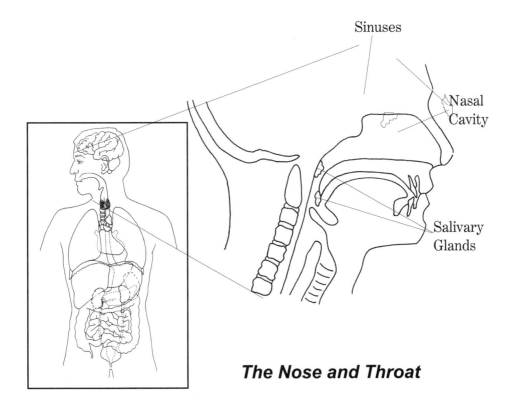

Sinuses

Nasal Cavity

Salivary Glands

The Nose and Throat

LUNGS/BRONCHIAL

The upper chest cavity protects the lungs, bronchi, bronchioles, and heart. The respiratory system provides the body with oxygen and carries off the carbon dioxide or waste product of the cells. The blood becomes enriched with oxygen. The degree to which this takes place can affect our energy level. A good practice is to breathe deep and expand the lungs.

The lungs work like bellows. They draw in air and force it out on regular intervals.

The diaphragm is a thin membrane that separates the upper chest cavity from the lower abdominal area. A diaphragm in spasm is very painful.

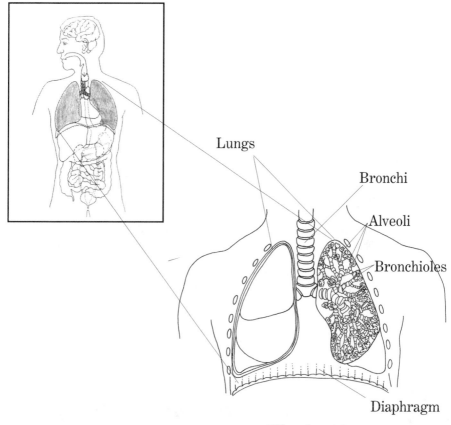

The Lungs

HEART

The heart is in the upper chest cavity and is protected by the rib cage. The heart is about the size of your clinched fist. As the heart beats it pushes the blood through myriads of arteries, capillaries, and veins. As the blood is pumped through the system, it carries food to the cells, and cell waste away. The heart has four chambers. (See figure below). There are valves between each of these chambers. A thin sac surrounds the heart. The sinoatrial node is located in the right atrial wall just below the superior vena cava. It initiates each heartbeat and is therefore called the "pacemaker."

Blood fresh with oxygen is brought to the heart through the pulmonary vein to the left atrium. The mitral valve opens to let blood into the left ventricle. The mitral valve prevents back flow of blood as it is pumped through the aortic valve to the body.

The aorta divides into smaller arteries; these branch into smaller blood vessels called arterioles, which connect into smaller capillaries. Food and oxygen are exchanged for waste products from the cells through the thin walls of the capillaries.

The waste products are carried away from the cells by small veins which become large veins and blood is returned to the right atrium of the heart via the superior and inferior vena cava. It flows through the tricuspid valve into the right ventricle. The tricuspid closes and blood is now pumped through the pulmonary valve into the lungs.

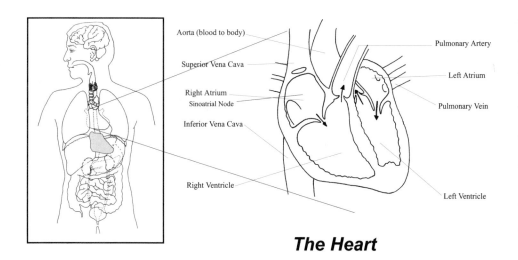

The Heart

LIVER/GALLBLADDER

The liver is the body's largest gland. The word "liver" comes from a Greek word meaning, "Life Giver." It lies just under the rib cage on your right side. The liver has been referred to as the chemical plant of the body and has the ability to regenerate itself. Bile is one of the substances manufactured by the liver and aids in digestion. Bile is stored in the gallbladder until it is ready for release during digestion into a section of the intestines called the duodenum.

Along with secretion of bile, the liver is important in the metabolism of carbohydrates, which helps maintain blood sugars, metabolism of fats and protein, removal of drugs and hormones, storage of certain vitamins, destroys worn out red and white blood cells, and activates formation of vitamin D.

The liver seems to be one of the first places you will find disease. If someone has a virus, bacteria, or allergy in the body, it usually shows up in the liver.

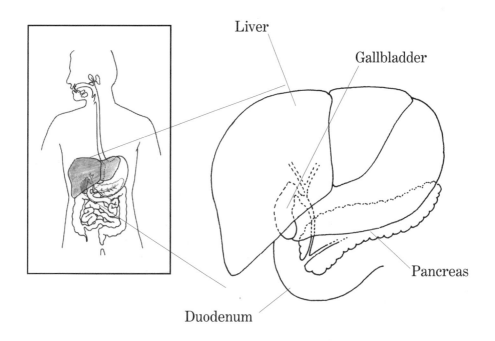

Liver

Gallbladder

Pancreas

Duodenum

STOMACH

Digestion begins in the mouth where food is mixed with saliva. From the mouth it moves through the esophagus into the stomach. The stomach secretes pepsin that continues the work of digestion. The stomach will vary in size, depending on the contents, and lies just below the diaphragm.

Food reaches the stomach, causing it to stretch, which stimulates nerves in the stomach to send messages to the brain to release gastric juices. There are those who advocate small frequent meals instead of three huge meals a day for those interested in weight maintenance. This would make sense for it keeps the stomach from getting too stretched out of shape. The bigger the stomach, the more food it requires to feel satisfied.

The stomach churns and mixes the food before passing it along through the small intestines.

A hiatal hernia is caused by the stomach trying to push up into the chest cavity. This can cause shortness of breath, shooting pains across the chest, gastric backwash, a "flip-flop" feeling in the chest, food to stick in the esophagus under the breastbone when swallowed, nausea, and a feeling of "fullness."

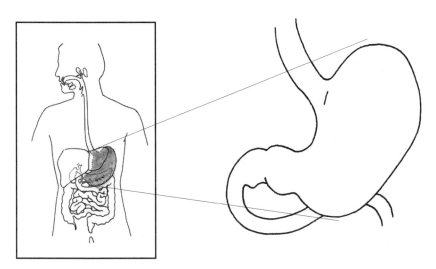

The Stomach

PANCREAS

The pancreas is located just below the rib cage extending from the right to about the middle of your upper abdominal area. It is shaped like a feather duster. The pancreas manufactures insulin and pancreatic fluid. Pancreatic fluid flows into the duodenum through a pancreatic duct.

Insulin is produced by a special group of cells within the pancreas called the islands of langerhans. Insulin is secreted directly into the blood stream. Insulin is necessary for the body tissues to utilize glucose, which is their form of fuel.

The pancreas is a deciding factor in such things as hypo/hyperglycemia and diabetes.

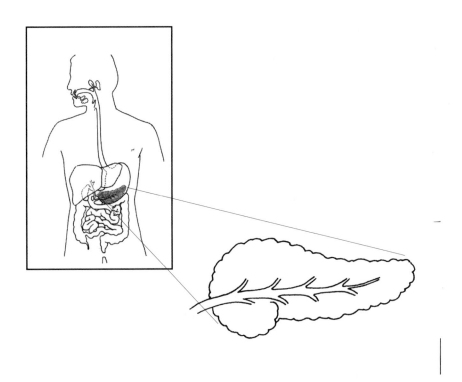

The Pancreas

SMALL INTESTINE

Food passes from the stomach into the small intestine. Here the digestion process continues. The small intestine is highly adapted for digestion and absorption of food. It has tiny villi that line the walls and ingest food as well as a long circular fold that allows time for absorption.

The small intestine is about an inch in diameter and can be about 10 feet long in an average adult. The small intestine is divided into three sections: the duodenum, the jejunum, and the ileum. The ileum lies between the small and large intestines. There is a valve between them that keeps food from flowing back from the large into the small intestine. It is called the ileocecal valve. This valve sometimes gets stuck open. If this happens, it can cause ringing in the ears, nausea, and pain in the appendix area.

Digested material is absorbed into the bloodstream from the small intestine. The waste, or bulk, is passed on into the large intestine. The action that moves food through the alimentary or digestive tract is called peristalsis.

The small intestine is a good site for parasite growth. Tapeworms are especially fond of this area. Ulcers in the duodenum are not uncommon.

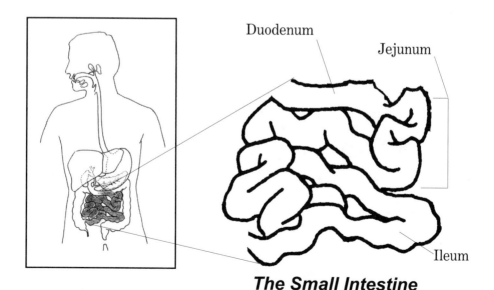

The Small Intestine

LARGE INTESTINE (COLON)

The large intestine is divided into three parts: the ascending, the transverse and the descending colon. The ascending section goes from the ileum of the small intestine up to mid abdominal area. The intestine then curves from right to left across the body just below the naval. This is called the transverse colon. The last section that curves and goes down on the left side of the body, ending in the rectum, is the descending colon.

Attached to the large intestine at the right lower quadrant is the appendix.

It is very important to eat foods high in fiber to keep the large intestine clear and moving.

Along the walls of the colon are nerve endings relative to every area of the body.

Food remains in the large intestine 3 to 10 hours. During this time the usable food material is absorbed. The rest becomes feces and is expelled through the rectal opening.

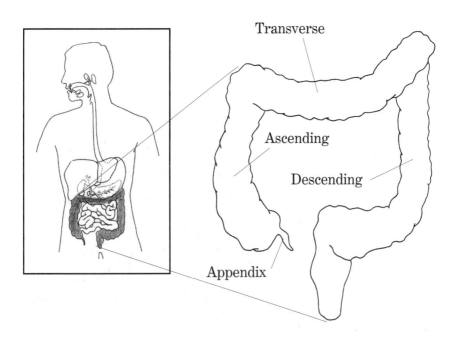

The Large Intestine

NERVOUS SYSTEM

The nervous system stems from the brain and is housed in the protective bones that make up the backbone. Nerves extend from the spinal chord and branch out to the various parts of the body in corresponding areas. Pinched nerves along the spinal column can cause weakened nerve impulses to internal organs. Infection, allergy, trauma or stress in the nervous system can be a contributing factor to feelings of nervousness, anxiety, depression, fibromyalgia, headache, and irritability that many people experience.

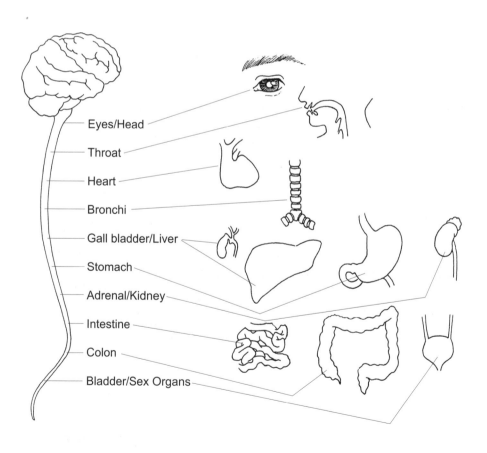

Eyes/Head

Throat

Heart

Bronchi

Gall bladder/Liver

Stomach

Adrenal/Kidney

Intestine

Colon

Bladder/Sex Organs

The Nervous System

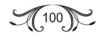
LYMPHATIC SYSTEM/SPLEEN

The lymphatic system is commonly known as the "second circulatory system" of the body. It is comprised of lymph nodes, tubes that run between these nodes, and small projections that reach into the cells to remove their waste products. Much like a sewage treatment plant, these nodes collect and destroy impurities, changing them so they can be issued out of the body through the skin, respiration, kidneys, or elimination process.

If the lymph nodes get overloaded or do not get the right amount of stimulation to function, impurities will remain in the body.

Lymphatic nodes full of infection are referred to as a "systemic infection." The flow of lymphatic fluid is enhanced with muscular contraction and deep breathing (another reason for strenuous physical exercise).

The spleen is the largest single mass of lymphatic tissue in the body.

The spleen is located just under the rib cage on the far left side of your body and is about the size of your heart. The spleen's main purpose is to store blood. The spleen also produces antibody plasma cells, destroys worn out blood cells, and helps in blood cell formation.

A swollen spleen is vulnerable to rupture if it gets hit very hard. The spleen is one of the first places Epstein-Barr will settle in the body.

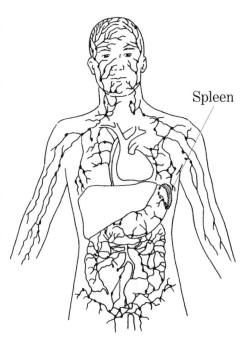

Spleen

The Lymphatic System/Spleen

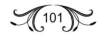

KIDNEYS/ADRENAL/URETER/BLADDER

Normally we have two kidneys, two ureters, a bladder, and a urethra. The function of this system is to secrete urine, which is a waste product of the cells carried to the kidneys by the blood.

The kidneys are bean shaped and sit next to the spine just about waist level. The ureters carry urine to the bladder. From the bladder, urine is expelled through the urethra.

Urine volume is influenced by blood pressure. Temperature, diuretics, mental state, and general health all play a part in the production of urine. Normal urine is sterile. It contains no disease-producing agents.

Tests done on urine can determine any number of physical diseases.

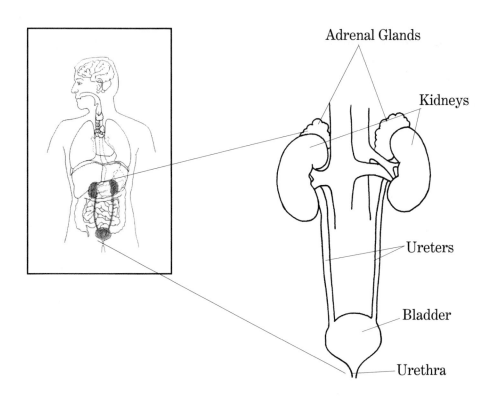

The Urinary System

FEMALE REPRODUCTIVE ORGANS

The female reproductive system is composed of the following organs: the ovaries, the fallopian tubes, the uterus, and the vagina.

The ovaries are about the size of an almond and contain thousands of eggs. When a baby girl is born, all the eggs she will ever have are already contained in her ovaries. During puberty, the eggs begin to ripen and are released to travel down the fallopian tubes to the uterus. If an egg unites with the male sperm, it is called fertilization. The egg will implant in the uterus where it begins rapid reproduction to become a baby in about nine months.

If the egg is not fertilized, it is taken from the uterus and right out of the body via the vaginal canal. Two weeks later the bloody lining that built up in preparation for pregnancy sloughs off. This is called the monthly cycle or menstruation.

This is repeated every month from puberty until the time of menopause.

Included in the female reproduction are the breasts. They respond to hormones during pregnancy and nursing. The mammary glands are important in the secretion of milk for the newborn infant.

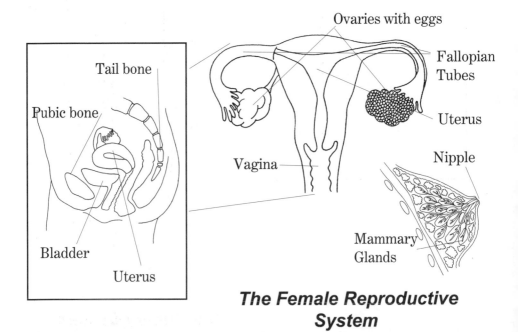

The Female Reproductive System

MALE REPRODUCTIVE ORGANS

The male reproductive organs consist of the scrotum, two seminal vesicles, ducts for spermatozoa, the prostate gland, and two bulbourethral glands.

The scrotum contains the testes, which produce the male sex hormones and spermatozoa. Sperm travels from the scrotum to the seminal vesicle where it is stored. When fluid is added to the sperm, it is called semen. Fluid is added at the seminal vesicle, by the prostate gland, and two small glands below the prostate called the bulbourethral glands.

The male penis contains the urethra, which is the external opening. The urethra is the passageway for urine and seminal fluid.

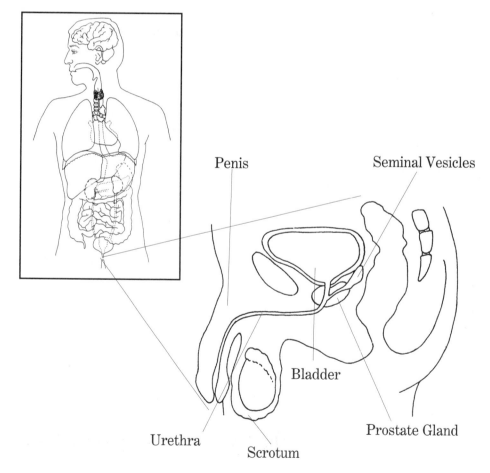

Penis   Seminal Vesicles

Bladder

Urethra   Prostate Gland

Scrotum

The Male Reproductive System

THYROID/PARATHYROID

The thyroid gland is located just above the top of the breast bone at the indented part of the throat.

The thyroid secretes hormones that regulate metabolism, growth and development, and the activity of the nervous system. This hormone is also a factor in the breakdown and excretion of cholesterol. Conditions that increase the body's need for thyroid hormones are cold environment, high altitude, and pregnancy. Aging slows down the thyroid, which is one of the determinants in weight gain as people age. The thyroid affects the sex organs, and in reverse, if the uterus or prostate is weak, it could have a negative influence on the thyroid.

Parathyroid glands are attached to the back of the thyroid gland. The parathyroid glands control the level of calcium and phosphate in the blood.

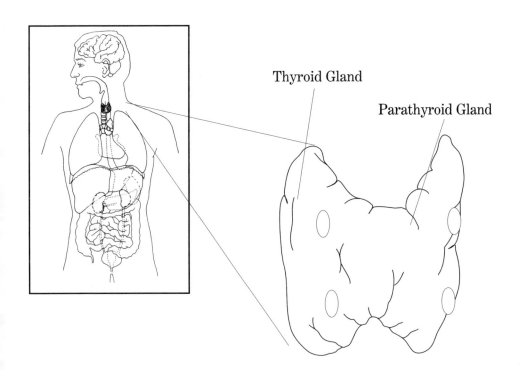

Thyroid Gland

Parathyroid Gland

The Thyroid/Parathyroid Glands

THYMUS

The thymus gland is directly behind the sternum, more commonly known as the breast bone, and rests between the lungs.

Medical science has determined that the thymus gland has some effect on growth, and is involved with the strength of muscular contraction and flow of lymph throughout the body. The thymus takes lymph cells from bone marrow and matures them to fight disease, which cells are now called "T Cells". It then secretes a hormone that trains and works with the T-Cells. The mature T-Cells are trained to go to an area of need where they pick up on unfamiliar cells and destroy them.

The thymus tends to shrink under continued stress. It is the link between mind and body and is the first organ affected by mental attitudes and negative experiences.

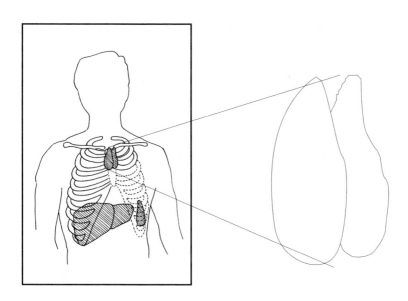

Thymus

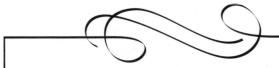

"If there is light in the soul,
There will be beauty in the person.
If there is beauty in the person,
There will be harmony in the house.
If there is harmony in the house,
There will be order in the nation.
If there is order in the nation,
There will be peace in the world."

— *Chinese Proverb*

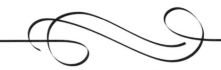

CHAPTER 7

Troubleshooting and the Thymus

The thymus regulates the movement of the meridian system. The thymus is located in the area of the heart chakra, which is the crossroad for the flow of energy as it passes from head to foot.

You might say the thymus is like the control room of a large energy plant sending energy where it is needed.

There is a continuous current of energy from one meridian point to another unless disease or injury occurs. If the energy flow is disrupted the corresponding organ will be weakened. Bio-Kinetic testing picks up on organ deficiencies since it works off the energy of the body.

Illness begins with a weakening or lessening of life's forces somewhere in the body, and can have its basis in any of the four areas of health which are physical, emotional, spiritual, or mental health.

The thymus gland is very sensitive to emotions.

Negative	Positive
Hate	Love
Envy	Faith
Suspicion	Trust
Fear	Courage
Anger	Gratitude
Jealousy	Cheerfulness

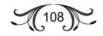

Positive thinking and a smiling face, whether seen on the human vista or simply drawn on a piece of paper, give a positive strength to the thymus gland. A smile brings cheer and strengthens the thymus!

THINGS THAT STRENGTHEN THE THYMUS:

- Pat on the back

- Nod of the head

- Outstretched arms in an embrace

- "Thumbs Up" sign

- Colors

- Wholesome music

- Pets

- Warm hugs

- Long walks on the beach

- Meditation

- Breathing mountain air

- Prayers and scriptures

The list is endless as we begin to look for the good.

You have an impact on other's health by the way you touch, talk to, look at, or respond to them.

The most important place to practice strengthening everyone's thymus is in the family and/or home. To have healthy children, it helps to provide positive emotions for their thymus.

When even one person raises his total health, everyone around is affected. Positive energy is reciprocated and everyone benefits.

THINGS THAT WEAKEN THE THYMUS:

- Advertisements that offend you

- Pornography

- Violence

- Loud offensive music

- Mean expressions

- Negative gestures

- Destructive drinks like alcoholic beverages and caffeine

- Tobacco products

- Drugs

- Insincere speakers from a platform or pulpit

- Unkind voices

- Any negative influence

- Allergies and Disease—you will learn to test for these with Bio-Kinetics in a later chapter.

Recognize the negative and remove whatever is possible from your life. Total health is enhanced when we are surrounded with positive images and positive feedback.

The thymus is strengthened through a simple technique: With your fingertips, tap lightly or rub the breastbone in small circular motions, starting at the throat area and going clockwise down the breastbone to the solar plexis (see diagram on following page). Or, you can simply tap over the area of the thymus gland.

This may be done several times a day.

When you begin testing and you find you are getting nothing but "Yes" or "No" to every question, have the person you are working on tap his thymus lightly, and you can do the same as you demonstrate to him where the thymus gland is located. This increases the positive energy flow in both of you.

The thymus gland in children is well developed and seems to shrink away as aging takes place. Perhaps this is because children have need of a healthy functioning immune system until childhood diseases are well behind them.

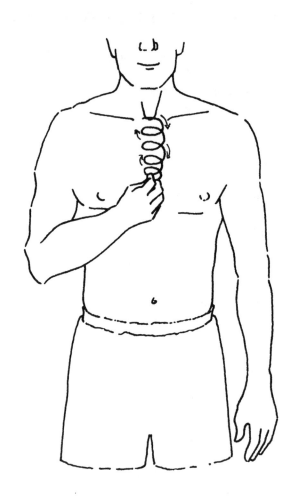

Strengthening the Thymus
With fingertips rub it gently in small
clockwise circular motions downward
beginning at the top of the breast bone.

The thymus can be encouraged at ANY AGE to continue to work for us. It is like the foreman in a factory. After all, even a foreman in a factory appreciates a pat on the back to encourage him on in his labors.

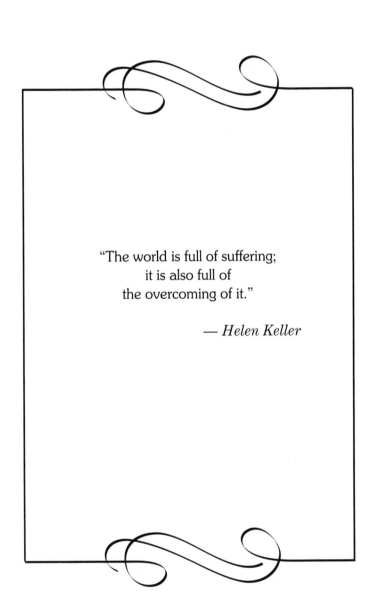

"The world is full of suffering;
it is also full of
the overcoming of it."

— *Helen Keller*

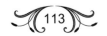

CHAPTER 8

Let's Test

With a basic understanding of the body, you are ready to begin the process of developing the skills needed to perform Bio-Kinetic testing.

As I mentioned earlier, BE PATIENT. The testing skill will come as you practice, study and hold firm to your desire to learn.

Bio-Kinetic testing utilizes the electrical impulses or energy of the Chinese meridians and chakra. Each body organ emanates energy. By directing your energy to the organs and asking certain questions, then swinging the hands or knees, you will get a noticeable response from that organ.

Kinesiology is a form of testing that requires resistence against a muscle of the body.

The difference between Bio-Kinetic testing and Kinesiology is that Bio-Kinetics does not use resistence or force.

This section will explain three methods of testing with Bio-Kinetics.

When testing is done between two people with a third person taking notes, you can compare it to using a computer: the person being tested is like the hard drive of the computer where all the information is stored; the one doing the testing represents the monitor that gets the informtion out where it can be seen and dealt with; and the note taker is the "printer." This is a full information system at your fingertips!

HOLDING A PRODUCT

This method utilizes the flow of energy over one of the chakra points.

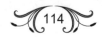
Any product you wish to know about can be held and tested.

The first thing to do is to find the chakra that works best for you. To do this, hold a product in the right hand and place the product directly over a chakra site. Now put the left hand over the top of the right hand with the product right next to the body.

The heart chakra (as mentioned earlier), is the center of energy and is the most commonly used site.

You may prefer to use the navel or throat chakra.

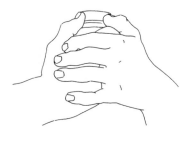

Hold product in right hand up to the chosen chakra site. Place left hand over right hand with product next to the body.

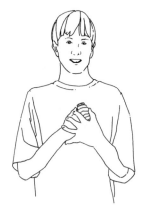

Heart

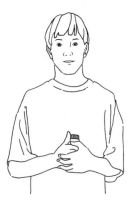

Navel

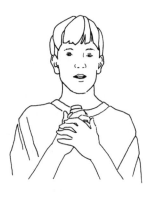

Throat

Standing in a relaxed position with your feet a few inches apart, ask your own energy, "Is this a good product for me?"

You should either sway forward or backwards. If you do *not* sway forward or backward, it means either 1) the product is not a positive or a negative, you have spent money on something that neither hurts nor helps you. Or, it means 2) you are not testable. To find out, tap the thymus and try another product.

If you sway this time, you are now able to test. Start again and ask the question, "Is this a good product for me?"

If you tip to the side or are pulled off balance, it means you are using the wrong chakra for your energy. Try placing the product over another chakra and ask the same question: "Is this a good product for me?"

If you are holding the product over the right chakra sight for you, then swaying forward is an affirmative or "Yes", this product is good for you.

Swaying backward is a negative or "No", this product is not good for you.

This is a good way to test products in a store or market. Testing a product will help you determine which brand is best. There are myriads of products on the market. Test different brands to get a feel for the energy pull of each one.

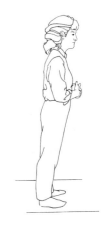

In holding the product over the right chakra, you find yourself swaying forward when you ask, "Is this a good product for me?", the answer is yes.

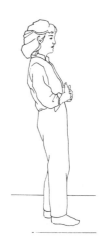

In holding the product over the same chakra site, you find yourself swaying backward when you ask, "Is this a good product for me?", the answer is no.

The three responses from products are:

1. A POSITIVE (pulled in a forward motion), which means that particular product will vibrate well with your energy to promote healing and health;

2. A NEGATIVE (swaying backwards), means you would not like how you feel with this in your body. It may cause headaches, rash, nausea, dizziness, or any number of allergic type reactions;

3. A NOTHING (standing without moving one way or another), indicates this product will neither hurt nor help, but would be a waste of money since it probably would simply flush through the system. Why spend money on a product that gives this response?

This form of testing is invaluable because it saves buying something, getting it home and finding out too late it is not for you. The obvious POSITIVE is known right there in the store.

Other questions that can be asked about a product while holding it:

"Would something else be better?"

"Can I use this in combination with my medicine?"

"How many capsules (or tablets) do I need?"

After asking this question, count slowly from one to ten. The right number of capsules will pull you forward and when you get to the amount that is not the right one, you will begin to sway backwards.

This method of testing for amounts is not as fast as the next two methods I will discuss. I prefer to use this method mostly to determine which brand is best. When I get home, I use another method to test for amount or strength of the product.

TESTING FOR AMOUNTS OF THE PRODUCT

If you choose to use this method for testing amounts, this is how it is done:

Holding the product over a chakra, ask the question: "Do I need one?" (Not moving) "Two?" (Not moving). "Three?" (swaying forward). This means three is the amount needed at the time.

Or, "Do I need one?" (Not moving). "Two?" (Not moving) "Three?" (Not moving) "Four?" (Swaying backwards). The last number that received a POSITIVE response is the best one. The response will either be moving forward into the POSITIVE position or backwards into the NEGATIVE.

I think what determines the direction is related to left and right brain strengths, thymus and health, or clarity of thought.

TESTING ON THE KNEES

This testing is done by:

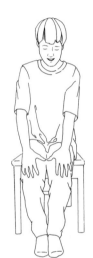

1. Sitting in a comfortable position with your legs forward on a chair. You want the whole upper part of the thighs to swing freely with the buttocks barely sitting on the chair.

2. Place your feet close together. The feet touching is best unless your thighs are too big to allow this position. If this is the case, the feet can be placed just outside the imaginary line from the knees to the floor about 16 inches apart.

3. Rest each hand on its corresponding knee cap.

4. Relax the shoulders and upper arms.

5. The forearm and hands will more than likely rest on the legs, or the arms can be held up so they form a straight line to the kneecap.

Illustration A
Sit comfortably on a chair with upper part of thighs able to swing freely and feet together. Hands are resting on each kneecap with thumbs extended straight together pointing inside.

How the arms fit on the legs and knees will be determined by the length of your arms. If you can barely reach your knees with your hands, hold your arms up off your legs. If you have long arms, it will not be like the picture, but your arms will actually rest on the upper part of your thigh. Either way is fine.

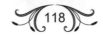

6. Extend your thumbs STRAIGHT together to the inside of your knees, with the thumbs pointed towards each other, as pictured in Illustration A.

7. Let your knees fall naturally apart, as shown in Illustration B.

Now, move your legs together by utilizing the strength in the legs and watch your thumbs.

Do they line up or go out of alignment?

Thumbs touching indicates a "Yes." If they go off to either side of each other or to the top or bottom, this is a "No".

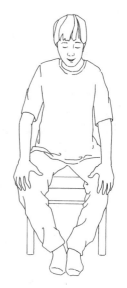

Illustration B
Let knees fall naturally apart.

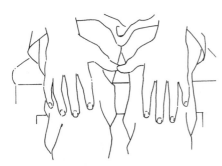

Thumbs lining up

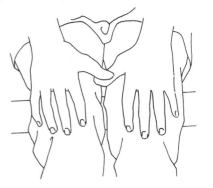

Thumbs out of alignment

This position can be used to test products, body parts, and anything else you wish to test.

TESTING WITH TWO PEOPLE

This form of testing is a merging of two energies. It also takes more muscular strength. The feet need to be held and swung to get responses.

It is interesting to me that those personalities who are gregarious or sociable do very well with this form of testing. Those who tend to be more independent or don't need people as much for survival do better testing on their own knees.

This position is not possible if you live alone or have no one around to test with.

Two people are needed: One to be tested while the other one does the testing.

The person being testing should be in a comfortable yet accessible position where the one doing the testing holds the feet and swings them freely.

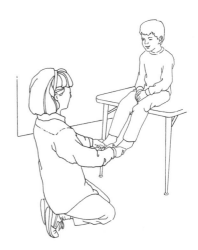

With this method of testing, different positions are possible. The person being tested could be lying on the floor with his head on a pillow, in which case the feet and legs need to be lifted right off the floor and swung together; he could be sitting on a table, counter or bench with the one doing the testing kneeling or sitting at his feet; or, a baby can be tested when he is asleep by gently lifting his feet and swinging them together.

One possible way to do a two person test.

Refer to the pictures for hand positions.

What to watch for when testing with the feet:

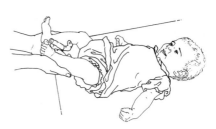

1. Place both hands so you can firmly grasp the ankles. If your client is lying down the feet need to be lifted

Testing a baby

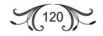

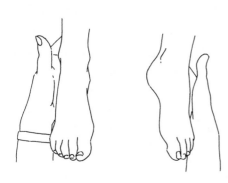

Illustration C
Lift and swing feet together.

and swung together, as shown in Illustration C. Or firmly grasp the toes if he is sitting on a table or bench with the feet dangling over the side, as shown in Illustration D. Your thumbs should be pointing straight towards each other on the inside of the feet.

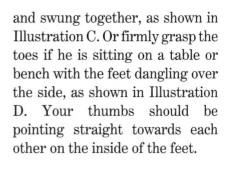

Illustration D
Place hands firmly on toes with thumbs pointing straight towards each other on inside of feet.

With your hands in this position, watch your thumbs to see if they go off alignment when you swing the feet together

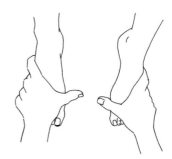

Thumbs out of alignment

or if they are perfectly lined up with each question asked.

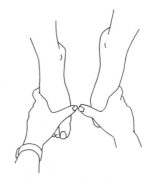

Thumbs perfectly aligned

2. If you find it hard to determine whether your thumbs are lined up or not, bend your thumbs down and draw a line up and down (as pictured) across the knuckle with a pen or water marker.

    Line the thumbs up and put them together gently to get the pen or marker rubbed off on the opposite thumb, then mark it more clearly with the marker.

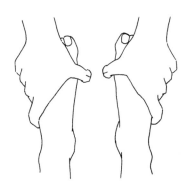

Testing with marked thumbs

After marking the thumbs, bend them down inside the feet instead of pointing them straight together. Now swing the feet and watch for the pen marks to line up or go off the mark.

3. Another option is to use stocking heel lines if they are available on the socks.

    When sock lines are used, please note that the feet need to be slightly twisted outward at the ankle so you can see the marks better. Hold the feet gently in both hands with the thumb over the top of the foot giving a slight twisting motion.

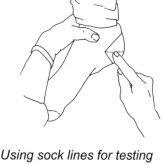

Using sock lines for testing

When you swing the feet watch for the sock marks to line up, or pull off the mark.

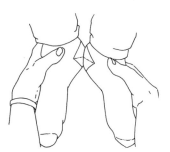

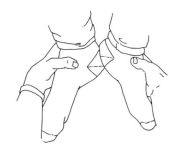

Sock marks line up   *Sock marks out of alignment*

4. It is also possible to mark the heels with a water soluble marking pen.

    Draw a straight short line on one heel in a perpendicular direction.

    This line will be the guide. Swing the feet together so they are even and make a mark on the corresponding heel.

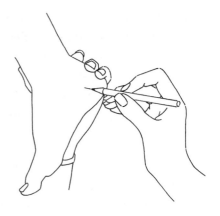

Drawing line on feet for measurement

These marks should line up and show the slightest deviation in the testing.

To be successful with this, make sure the marks are exactly opposite each other.

Swing the feet and see if the marks go off alignment . . .

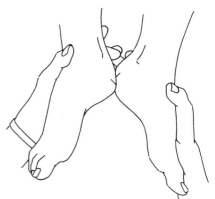

Heel marks out of alignment

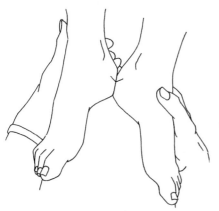

. . . or if they line up perfectly.

Heel marks perfectly aligned

5.   Hold the heels in the palms of your hands. Holding both hands in a cupping shape, let his feet rest in the cup formed by the palm of your hands, as illustrated.

Now, extend the index fingers so they come together straight as arrows. Keep them straight, not letting them bend upwards, or the reading will be off.

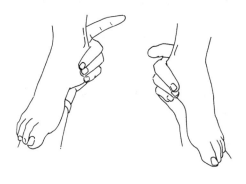

Holding heels in palms of hands

Look down between the feet and watch for the fingers to line up or go off mark.

It is advisable to learn all methods of testing. You never know when a different method will work better.

Whatever position you choose to use, IT IS IMPORTANT TO HAVE FREE MOVEMENT WITHOUT FRICTION. Be aware that dragging the legs or feet on the floor or a chair will throw the testing off. It makes one side pull unevenly.

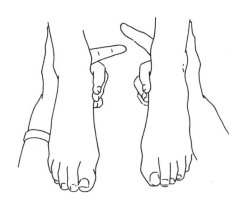

Extending index fingers going off mark

THE PERSON BEING TESTED SHOULD TOTALLY RELAX HIS LEGS. Any tightening or jerking of his legs or feet will negatively affect the test. Everyone wants to be a helper, but now is NOT the time.

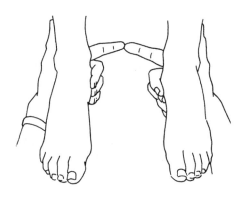

Fingers lining up

THE FIRST QUESTION

Having established which position is most comfortable and easy to use, let's begin.

Sit or kneel with your back straight and arms extended, keep a firm but soft hold on the person's feet you are testing, or sit with your hands on your knees.

Relax and take a deep breath.

Ask a question to begin with that will verify that you are testing properly; a question you already know the answer to, like your name or the name of the person you are testing, is a good beginning.

Say the questions out loud at first. As you begin to feel more comfortable with the testing, you will be able to ask the questions in your mind.

"Is your name ('my name' if you are testing yourself) _____?" (Ask the first given name).

> Slowly bringing the feet or knees together. Watch for the thumbs, marks, or lines (hereafter referred to as INDICATORS) to come together. They should line up on this question with a POSITIVE response.

> > If they do not line up, tap the thymus or try a different position.

> > > Swing the feet or knees again and watch for a response from the INDICATORS. If you are testing correctly, they should now line up.

Next, ask a name you know is NOT the correct one:

"Is your name ('My name' if you are testing yourself) Rupunzel?"

> Slowly bring the feet together. Watch for the INDICATORS to go off alignment. They should NOT come together on this question. Move the feet slowly at first to get a feel for the swinging motion.

> > An incorrect answer will cause the INDICATORS to go off with a NEGATIVE response.

Practice asking the name a few times until you feel comfortable with the flow of energy directing your response.

HOW DOES THIS WORK?

Your energy knows what is truth or error.

When an *untruth* is projected into the energy field it causes the muscles to contract. This action pulls the muscles into a negative response or out of alignment, in the INDICATORS.

If the question is *truth,* the muscles will stay relaxed and will come together without resistence. This gives a positive response, or perfect alignment as seen through the INDICATORS.

THE "OUT," "IN," OR "OKAY," WORD

The next thing to establish is the word you are most comfortable with to help determine the response via the INDICATORS.

The choice of words most often used are "OUT," "IN," or "OKAY".

USING OUT

I, personally, use the word "OUT" because I am interested in finding those things that indicate something is wrong so I can test for what is needed to correct the weakness.

When the indicators line up or show a positive response with the word "OUT," it means, "Yes, it has something wrong with it. Yes, It is OUT."

If the INDICATORS go off or are negative, it means, "NO, it is not out and is perfectly okay".

If you are a personality type who cannot stand to have anything out of order, this would not be the best choice of a word for you. In your mind, you would tend to reject the notion that something might be "out of place."

In that case, the words "IN" or "OKAY" would be better.

USING IN OR OKAY

If these words are used, the response would be opposite of the "OUT" word. INDICATORS lined up means "Yes, it is healthy or the right product". INDICATORS off means, "It is NOT okay. Something is wrong and needs to be tested further."

To clarify this, just remember that INDICATORS lined up is ALWAYS a YES no matter what word you use. It means, "Yes, it is OUT," or "Yes, it is IN."

To find which word you are most comfortable with, I will walk you through a test on the neck bones.

"Is your (my) neck OUT?" Swing the feet or knees together and watch the INDICATORS.

YES or positive means "Yes, the bones are out."

If the INDICATORS do not line up, it means, "No, the bones are NOT out of alignment and are healthy."
OR
"Is your (my) neck IN?" Swing the feet or knees together and watch the INDICATORS.

A YES or positive response means "Yes, the bones are IN or healthy."

INDICATORS off, or in a negative position means, "No, the bones are not in, or are not healthy."

It is important to swing his feet apart, then stop and ask the question BEFORE you begin bringing the feet or knees together. This gives the brain a chance to direct the energy and get a message to the muscles.

Think of one question at a time or the brain will be moving on to the next question and you will not get the right response. Always start slow. You can pick up speed as you practice and get better asking the questions.

Another thing I have found beginners tend to do is "pump" the feet of the one they are testing. Hold the feet absolutely still as the brain thinks of the question, then bring the feet slowly together.

Word and Indicator Meaning Table

	ON thumbs, lines or indicators match up	OFF thumbs, lines or indicators don't match up
OUT	Not healthy, not right choice of product, not in alignment, has something wrong with it	It is healthy, nothing is wrong
OKAY/IN	Yes, it is okay	No, something is wrong

Indicators lining up ALWAYS mean YES . . . . Yes, something is wrong, Yes, it is fine, Yes, it is OKAY.

TESTING THROUGH A PROXY

There are situations where it is not possible to deal directly with the person needing the testing. Some of the possible circumstances are as follows:

Situation: A child is so wiggly it is impossible to test by holding on to her feet.

Situation: Someone lives away from you and needs to be tested.

Situation: Someone has a leg or foot amputated.

Situation: You have a hard time testing someone through his feet.

How is the testing done when these situations arise? We use a proxy.

Testing through a proxy means using someone else's feet or your own knees to do the testing for another person.

To help explain how this is possible, let's use electricity as an example.

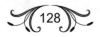

If a group of people were standing together holding hands, and the first person in line grabbed a hold of an electric fence, which person would get the shock? The person at the end of the line.

Electricity travels until it finds a way out.

The body's energy utilizes this same principle. When a proxy is used, the questions are sent through the proxy but pass right on to the person being tested—like they are the one at the end of the line of the electric fence analogy.

Your thoughts are sending energy to the one you wish to test.

When a proxy is used, it is important to get permission, or clearance, from both parties before continuing with the testing.

Ask these questions:

1. "Can I use you as a proxy for (fill in the name of the one being tested)?"

2. "Can I test you (name of the one being tested) through(name of proxy)?"

The person being tested does not have to be in the same room. Your energy will seek them out wherever they are.

I have had children travel and live in different states and countries. When I needed to test them I used a younger brother or sister they got along well with as the proxy.

Is it possible that you CANNOT test through the proxy? Yes. This will happen if there are any negative feelings between the proxy and the one being tested or if the proxy has some skepticism or misunderstanding about the testing you are about to do.

If this happens, admit that you are unable to use that person and find someone else to serve as proxy.

Negative feelings block the energy flow.

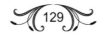

Using someone else's feet

Once you have permission to test through a proxy, place your hands in position on the proxy's feet, and you are ready to begin the test.

This is the format:

"Is it possible to test _____ through you?"

(At this point, you must totally concentrate on the one you wish to test. Visualize him in your mind. Think about him with each question.)

"Is _____'s neck out?"

Follow the format for testing an individual through the proxy, as if the individual you are testing were there with you. Swing the feet for each question you ask and watch the INDICATORS for a response.

TESTING THROUGH YOUR KNEES

If you decide to use your knees instead of another person as proxy, it is possible to use your own energy. When you use your knees, you become the proxy.

With the hands in place on your knees, fingers or thumbs directed to the inside, swing the knees for each question asked.

Following is the format:

"Can I use myself as a proxy for _____?"

"Can I test you _____ through me?"

"Is your neck out?"

Continue and ask each question.

Repeating the word "your" and mentally thinking about the one being tested will keep the energy directed to him instead of sending it back to you.

Swing the knees for each question asked.

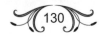

TESTING YOURSELF THROUGH A PROXY

Sometimes it is hard to test yourself drawing upon your own energy. If this happens, you will need someone else to test against.

If this is the case, you will be testing yourself through a proxy.

Using the feet of a proxy, swing the feet for each question and ask:

"Can I test myself through you?"

"Is my neck out?"

Notice in this situation you are using the word "my" and thinking about yourself and your body which pulls the energy through the proxy to you. The proxy becomes a mirror reflecting back to you questions you want to ask about yourself.

This is successful only if the proxy gives permission energy wise. I have seen situations where verbal permission was given in an attempt not to offend, but the energy knew the true feelings and did not really want to accommodate the one doing the testing.

The testing did not work!

I had a woman ask me once to test her son who was in a foreign country. I could not get through to him. I asked her a few questions and found out they had a terrible relationship. Her comment was, "He was the orneriest little snot. I was so glad when he left."

There was definitely a wall between them. This is something we always respect as healers. We never go where we are not invited or allowed to be.

If you are unable to test through the proxy, find someone else to serve as your proxy. It's as simple as that.

Follow the exact pattern for testing body parts, supplements, or other questions you may have about yourself, that will be outlined in the following chapter.

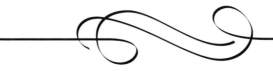

"If I can stop one heart from breaking,
I shall not live in vain;
If I can ease one life the aching,
Or cool one pain,
Or help one fainting robin
Unto his nest again,
I shall not live in vain."

— *Emily Dickinson*

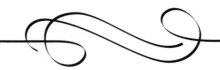

CHAPTER 9

Order For Testing

Now that you have laid the groundwork, you are ready to put the knowledge to work.

As you do the testing, I'd like for you to feel like I am right there by you. It is a thrill for me to see my students catch on to the testing and begin to use it. Therefore, know that I share in your excitement.

Be very patient and begin slowly at first.

General rule: Start at the top of the body and work down.

See the Bio-Kinetic checklist in the appendix at the back of the book.

I have devised a form that serves me well. My clients use this checklist to make their own notes and then take it home with them.

The material in this book is copyrighted. However, you do have permission to copy this page as well as the Epstein Barr/ Yeast cleansing diet page. I have spent years developing this method. My hope is to save you time as you begin your testing.

I suggest you go make a lot of copies of the checklist page and put one right next to you as you do your testing. Follow the format along as you go down through the different sections of testing.

I have divided the body into sections to help facilitate the memorization and testing of each organ. Committing as much as possible to memory will save you time when you begin testing.

Organizing the Body Into Sections Table

SECTION 1	SECTION 2	SECTION 3	SECTION 4
Neck	Brain	Nervous system	Pituitary
Back	Eyes	Lymphatic system	Thyroid
Upper	Ears	Spleen	Parathyroid
Mid	Nose	Kidneys	Thymus
Lower	Throat	Ureter	Pancreas
Hips	Lungs	Bladder	Adrenal
(Other Bones)	Bronchioles	Ovaries	
Muscles	Heart	Uterus	
Ligaments	Liver/Gallbladder	Prostate	
Tendons	Stomach	Blood system	
	Small Intestine		
	Large Intestine		

Section 1 are the bones and all the things connected with them.

Section 2 are the solid inner organs. Start with the head (brain), and EENT (eyes, ears, nose, throat), then the chest (heart, lungs, bronchioles), the stomach and liver, and finally the intestines.

Section 3 are the water organs. These are associated with body fluids. The spinal fluid in the nervous system, the lymphatic fluid, the urinary organs, the reproductive organs, and the blood stream.

Section 4 is the endocrine system. (The reproductive organs are also considered endocrine, but they are categorized under the "water" section for testing purposes.)

WALK THROUGH ON A BODY TEST

Choose a testing position you can work with.

Testing on another person.

"Is your name _____?" (Yes)

"Is your name Rupunzel?" (No)

"Are you testable?" (Yes)

"May I test you?" (Yes)

OUT   IN   OKAY

Section 1:

- "Is your neck out?"

- "Is your back out?"

- "Are your hips out?"

- "Are your muscles out?"

(I only test ligaments and tendons if there is a need.)

Reminder: Are you using the right word for you—out, in, or okay?

Section 2:

- "Is your brain out?" (Imagine the response when I ask this out loud.)

- "Are your eyes out?"

- "Are your ears out?"

- "Is your nose out?"

- "Is your throat out?"

- "Are your lungs out?"

- "Are your bronchioles out?"

- "Is your heart out?"

- "Is your liver/gallbladder out?"

- "Is your stomach out?"

- "Is your small intestine out?"

- "Is your large intestine out?"

Reminder: Are you asking the question BEFORE swinging the INDICATORS together? This keeps your mind focused.

Section 3:

- "Is your nervous system out?"

- "Is your lymphatic system out?"

- "Is your spleen out?"

- "Are your kidneys out?"

- "Are your ureters out?"

- "Is your bladder out?"

- "Are your ovaries out?" (Women only)

- "Is your uterus out?" (Women only)

- "Is your prostate out?" (Men only)

Reminder: Are you thinking about the person you are testing?

Section 4:

- "Is your pituitary out?"

- "Is your thyroid out?"

- "Are your parathyroids out?"

- "Is your pancreas out?"

- "Are your adrenals out?"

Reminder: Remember to bring the feet or the knees together slowly for each question.

Make a note of the negative responses you see via the INDICATORS. These are the organs you will want to concentrate on for further testing.

This is a complete body test.

It is not always necessary to test every organ. I do so when I am working with clients and they are making notes of the testing.

Other times, for instance, when a child says, "My head aches," I will get right to the point and ask, "Why does your head ache? Is it an infection? Stress? Trauma?"

It is not necessary to test the whole body to pinpoint the reason for headaches, jammed thumbs, or other complaints where you do not have the time to go through the whole body system.

An example of this was the time I was riding my bike past a park where my daughter was playing with some friends.

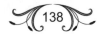

My daughter came running over to me and asked me to come quickly because her friend was hurt.

When I approached, I found the young lady lying in pain and unable to move. I was not concerned at the time whether she had a virus or allergies anywhere in her body. The concern then and there was whether she had broken any bones.

So, I asked the question, "Are your bones out?" Yes. "Are they broken?" Yes. "Is it the neck?" No. "Is it the shoulders?" No. "Is it the clavicle (collar bone)?" Yes. Is your back broken anywhere?" No.

It just took a few seconds to pinpoint the source of her pain. I also tested the muscles and found some pulled muscles.

In a case like this, there is a strong possibility of shock. I could tell from her body language that she might be in shock. It tested in the affirmative.

I sent her friends for some blankets and then elevated her feet. When her mother arrived on the scene, I recommended she call an ambulance because of the break I had detected.

When the paramedics arrived, they poked and asked questions and declared it to be a pulled muscle. They put a sling on her and helped her get to her mother's car, all with great pain and difficulty for the girl.

I thought nothing more about it until the next day when her mother called and said, "You were right. It was a broken collarbone. How did you know that?"

Did I need to do the complete body test at this time? No. You also will be able to test to whatever detail is needed under the circumstances you are in.

Tips for Testing

- **Avoid "pumping" the hands or feet as you test.** Hold your hands very still, as the question, then slowly bring the indicators together.

- **When you are testing someone, direct the question to the person you are testing.** For example, ask, "Are *your* eyes (etc.) in?" By asking, "Are his/her eyes out?" you are directing your energy to someone else. By using the word "your," the energy is sent directly to the one being tested.

- **The indicators do not have to be very far off.** For teaching purposes, the illustrations in the book show them being way off. If your indicators are off, even a small degree, they are still off. They may be off above or below or to either side. It is still *off.*

- **Avoid asking the same question over and over again.** It will confuse your energy. If you want to verify if something is wrong, ask the question in a different way. For example, ask, "Are you sure my bones are really out?"

- **Trust your answer.** Learn to respect the energy you are working with. Do not doubt that you have received information that is truth to you or the one you are testing. This is why you are learning bio-kinetic testing. You ask, and you will receive.

- **Get very specific with your questions.** Bio-Kinetics teaches you to become a detailed interrogator! When testing for a certain product at the store, ask more questions. For example: "Is this the best product there is for me?" "Would something in this store be better?" "In addition to what I already tested for, do I still need this product?" "Is there something in my home that I have that I could use for this problem?"

- **It is possible to test for food for the day.** Some days you will be able to eat a hamburger; another day you will test not to eat it. One day chocolate may be okay, while another day it would be upsetting to your energy. Things change on a continuum as the body is exposed to different elements, stresses and climate changes. Learn to test for everything you eat, drink, and take into your body.

It is not possible for me to anticipate every question and every need you may have. As you carefully test and tune in to the higher energy available to you, be wise, think through what it is you really want to know, then ask for it. Relax, enjoy, and be at peace with the knowledge you will receive.

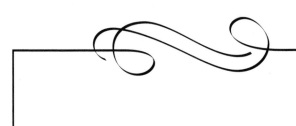

"All I have seen teaches me to
Trust the Creator for all
I have not seen."

— *Ralph Waldo Emerson*

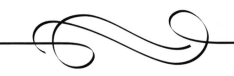

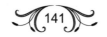

CHAPTER 10

And What Are We Testing For?

This is a basic guideline of the more common ailments you might expect to find.

As already stated, never try to diagnose something of a serious nature. Leave that to healthcare professionals.

If you do find something that may need medical attention, be open-minded to that fact and recommend a medical checkup.

With each of the body parts, I have listed different things that can be tested for. Swing the feet for each one listed.

The word "other" is at the end of each body part. There are always other ailments that exist that may be more of a medical nature. If you get a "YES" with the word "other" then decide from there where you need to go for the answer.

BONES: broken, out of alignment, infection, Epstein-Barr, bruised, jammed, fractured (hairline or major), arthritis, bursitis, gout, calcium deplete, calcium deposits, birth defect, growth plates, bone spurs, other

MUSCLES: allergies, bacteria, yeast, Epstein-Barr, virus, pulled, sprained, torn, herniated, other

BRAIN: allergies, yeast, Epstein-Barr, virus, mineral deposits, medicine storage, blood clot, stroke, bruised, parasites, stress, tumor, drugs, trauma from accident, other

EYES: allergies, bacteria, yeast, Epstein-Barr, virus, nearsighted, muscle weakness, farsighted, glaucoma, torn retina, eyestrain, other

EARS: allergies, bacteria, yeast, Epstein-Barr, virus, wax build-up, nerve damage, other

NOSE/THROAT: allergies, bacteria, yeast, Epstein-Barr, virus, herpes, sexually transmitted diseases, growths, esophageal reflux, cancer, medicine storage, other

LUNGS/BRONCHIOLES: allergies, bacteria, yeast, Epstein-Barr, virus, cancer, medicine storage, tuberculosis, other

HEART: bacteria, Epstein-Barr, virus, endocarditis, Pericarditis, weak muscle, weak valve, weak pacemaker, constricted arteries, constricted veins, congestive heart, other

LIVER: allergies, bacteria, yeast, Epstein-Barr, virus, parasites, medicine storage, hepatitis, mineral deposits, medicine storage, gallstones, radiation, cancer, drugs, other

STOMACH: allergies, bacteria, yeast, Epstein-Barr, virus, parasites, ulcer, hyper-acidic, hypo-acidic, hiatal hernia, medicine storage, valves not working, stress, cancer, radiation, other

SMALL INTESTINES: parasites (especially tapeworm), yeast, ulcer, other

LARGE INTESTINE: allergies, bacteria, yeast, Epstein-Barr, virus, parasites, ulcers, spastic colon, collapsed colon, fecal impaction, diverticulitis, appendicitis, ileocecal valve not shut, stress, cancer, other

NERVOUS SYSTEM: allergies, bacteria, yeast, Epstein-Barr, virus, trauma, stress, pinched nerves, drugs, other

LYMPHATIC SYSTEM: allergies, bacteria, yeast, Epstein-Barr, virus, radiation, medicine storage, cancer, other

SPLEEN: Epstein-Barr, medicine storage, ruptured, other

KIDNEYS: allergies, bacteria, yeast, Epstein-Barr, virus, stress, mineral deposits, medicine storage, drugs, stones, cancer, other

URETER/BLADDER: weak muscles, collapsed, virus, Epstein-Barr, yeast, bacteria, cancer, other

OVARIES: yeast, virus, Epstein-Barr, cysts, hormone storage, menopause, other

UTERUS: bacteria, yeast, Epstein-Barr, collapsed, hormone changes, hormone storage, sexually transmitted disease, pregnancy, growths, cysts, scar tissue, endometriosis, parasites, warts, cancer, other

PROSTATE: Epstein-Barr, swollen, cancer, sexually transmitted diseases, other

BLOOD SYSTEM: bacteria, yeast, Epstein-Barr, virus, parasites, anemia, leukemia, lupus, cancer, medicine storage, Ph balance out, electrolytes out of balance, other

PITUITARY: tumor, out of alignment, not secreting properly, other

THYROID: underactive, overactive, growths, cancer, goiter, radiation, other

PARATHYROID: growths, underactive, overactive, other

THYMUS: underactive

PANCREAS: hyperactive, hypoactive, Epstein-Barr, medicine storage, parasites, other

ADRENAL: stress, bruised, overactive, other

TESTING WHAT IS WRONG

The suggestions given to test body parts are only a guideline and cover the more common ailments. If there is something you do not understand, make

sure you seek competent medical help. Bio-Kinetic testing is limited only by individual knowledge.

I will walk you through a testing on the bones, following the suggested guideline above. All other organs will use the same pattern.

Swing the feet or knees for each question.

- "Is your name_____?"

- "Are you testable?"

- "Are your bones out?" (Yes)

- "Is it your neck?" (No)

- "Is it your upper back?" (Yes)

- "Is your back broken?" (No)

- "Is it out of alignment?" (Yes)

When you get an affirmative answer, that may be the only thing wrong, or it's possible there is something else on the list you need to check.

- "Is there anything else wrong with the bones?" (Yes)

- "Do you have an infection in the bones?" (No)

- "Are the bones bruised?" (No)

- "Are the bones jammed?" (No)

- "Is there a fracture in the bones?" (No)

- "Do you have arthritis?" (Yes)

- "Is there anything else wrong with the bones?" (No)

At this point I would decide that the bones were out of alignment and needed to have a chiropractic adjustment. Along with the misalignment, there is a showing of arthritis.

It is possible to check exactly which bone has the arthritis if you know the names of the bones.

Unless you really want to know, it's not vitally important as far as the testing goes to know which bone or bones the arthritis is in, because when you test for bone nutrients, it will be the same for all the bones. Bones cells vibrate to the same healing tools.

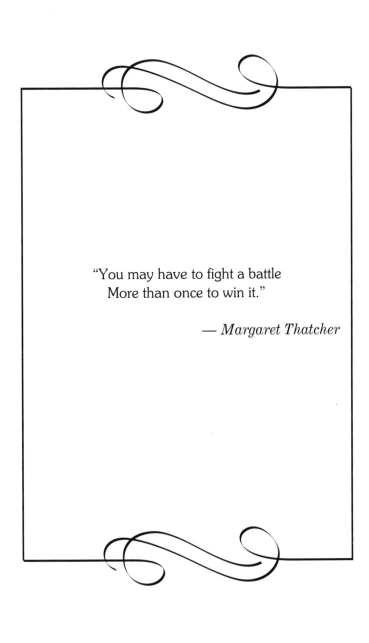

"You may have to fight a battle
More than once to win it."

— *Margaret Thatcher*

CHAPTER 11

Types of Infection

The body is constantly in a state of readiness, like an armed force at war, to combat outside invasions.

When these agents gain entrance into the body causing symptoms of pain, swelling, heat, fever, etc., then the invading force becomes an infection.

Even as you sit here and read this book, there are millions of immune cells coursing through your bloodstream looking for invading agents to "attack" and eat. Many of the immune cells actually ingest the infectious cell.

We have already discussed the immune system and the function of the thymus. Remember that emotional stress can upset the delicate balance and bring on a "stress illness."

During times of stress it is vital to give your body more nutrients which support the immune cells and give them strength to accomplish their job. Stress taxes your whole body. When you find yourself in a stressful situation, take a deep breath, then test for the nutrients you need to get you through the crisis.

Eat well, get plenty of rest, exercise, and increase your supplementation when you are experiencing a stress crisis.

A knowledge of healing, supplements, and relaxation techniques is good to have. They definitely give your body the edge in the ongoing battle against illness and disease.

You may have noticed when reading the section "And What Are We Testing For", that some common things kept showing up. These seem to be the main underlying causes of so many health complaints.

The five main culprits of illness are:

- Allergies

- Bacteria

- Yeast (Candida)

- Virus

- Parasites

Memorize these. You will become well acquainted with them. They will crop up constantly in your testing.

In order to understand more about them, I will explain a little bit about each one. Again, this is a very basic, tip-of- the-iceberg explanation. If you want to know more, there are many good resource books available. Places to look for information include health food stores, the local library, and college classes.

ALLERGIES

Allergies and the harm they do to the system is not generally understood.

There are many variables about allergies.

1. An allergy can be inherited.

2. Allergies can vary in type and severity even in the same family.

3. Allergies can come and go overnight.

4. Allergies can be made worse by another infectious agent.

5. Allergies can be to only one part of a food, not necessarily the whole food product. An example of this is milk. Is it the fat, the calcium, the lactose, or the enzymes in milk that you are allergic to?

6. Allergies have varying degrees of severity. Some are bad enough to cause death, while others are barely noticeable.

7. You may crave the allergy producing food, but more than likely you will say, "I always hated that and Mom made me eat it!" (And "No" this does not include the dislike children seem to have for vegetables!)

Once an allergy is in the system, it takes about two weeks to get it cleaned out. During this time, you need to stay away from the allergy-producing agent.

Some allergies are severe enough that they need to be absolutely avoided because they cause anaphylactic shock.

Anaphylactic shock is a sudden or violent sensation passing through the body strong enough to cause involuntary muscle contractions and depress body functions. This does not always, but has many times resulted in death. This type of shock is caused by an allergic reaction to an allergenic agent in the system.

This is the type of shock I experienced when I took the wrong kind of medicine for my body. You have read about this in my personal story.

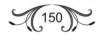

These allergy sufferers need only one incident to know they will watch that allergen for the sake of their life.

Some allergies can be overcome or outgrown. With Bio-Kinetic testing skills, you can determine whether this is possible.

Swing the feet and ask, "Can this allergy be overcome?" (Yes or No)

Following is a method I have used on our children and family members to help them overcome pollen, food, and chemical allergies.

Have your client lie down or sit in a comfortable position.

Using the Chinese meridian chart on page 31, swing the feet for each meridian and ask if it is weakened by the allergy.

Ask, "How many meridians are weakened by this allergy? One? Two? Three?" Counting until the INDICATORS go off or are negative.

This gives the number of meridians to watch for.

Then ask the question:

"Which ones are they? Is the heart meridian affected?" (No)

"Is the small intestine meridian affected?" (No)

"Is the bladder meridian affected?" (Yes)

Make a note of this one and continue the circle of meridians until the ones that are weakened give a positive test.

Look where the beginning and ending points are of the meridians. Tap gently on the beginning AND the end of each meridian point with two of your fingers. (I use the pointer and middle fingers).

The tapping is done in a waltz rhythm with the ONE count being harder than the next two: ONE two three, ONE two three, ONE two three, etc.

Have an assistant keep time for you or watch the clock while you do the waltz rhythm tapping for 30 seconds. It is easier if someone else is watching so you can concentrate on keeping your fingers in place on the meridian points.

After 30 seconds on those two points, go to the next meridian and repeat the process.

Ask your client to concentrate on the product he is being strengthened against.

For instance, if it is hay pollens, then he should visualize smelling new mown hay, running through it, rolling in it, etc.

If it's a food, he should imagine the taste, the smell, and the texture in his mouth.

After having the meridians reset against that allergy, he should stay away from it for two days. This is important.

Because you need to avoid the allergen for two days, this eliminates a few allergies from being reset if they are constantly in the air and being breathed.

I reset my son against cigarette smoke. We went to the movies before the two days were up and as we walked out someone was standing outside smoking. The minute we breathed the cigarette smoke I could sense the setback this was to my son's system.

When we got home I retested him. We went through the process again of resetting the meridians. It worked that time.

If you are resetting pollen allergies, wait until winter when the pollens are covered up with snow.

Food is easy to reset against because it can be avoided for two days by just not eating it.

Allergies come from four sources:

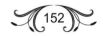

1. **Something you eat.** The most common food allergies are eggs, milk, chocolate, wheat, corn, nuts, fish, citrus foods, tomatoes, pesticide sprays and chemical additives.

2. **Something you breathe.** Breathing allergies are things such as pesticides, chemical pollutants, perfumes, petroleum-based products and exhaust, cigarette smoke, pollens, factory pollutants, soaps, shampoos, and some animal dander. In fact, anything you can imagine existing in the air someone will be allergic to.

3. **Something you touch.** Touching allergies would be plants, chemicals, animal dander, material, shampoos, or soaps (usually the allergy would be to the chemical or perfume base in the product).

4. **Something that bites you.** Insect allergies come from being bitten by various bugs or insects. Bee stings are an example of how allergies affect the body. You might be stung and swell up slightly, or suffer severe anaphylactic shock.

It is possible to have more than one allergy.

Be creative in allergy testing. Each individual is unique in their chemical make-up and allergic reactions.

Testing for allergies

After testing the body parts and finding an allergy, the format for testing for allergies is:

Swing the feet for each question.

-   "Are the allergies in your body to something you are eating?" (Yes)

-   "Is it eggs?" (No)

-   "Is it milk?" (Yes)

-   "Are you allergic to another food product?" (Yes)

-   "Is it chocolate?" (Yes)

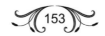

- "Are you allergic to anything else that you eat?" (Yes)

The list of foods seems endless. It helps to break it down into categories,

- "Is it a fruit?" (No)

- "Is it a vegetable?" (No)

- "Is it a grain?" (Yes)

Other categories could include:

- fungi and molds

- sprays

- chemicals

- MSG or flavorings

- preservative

- food colorings

Be creative in testing for food.

After determining that the food he is allergic to is a grain, think about the grain products and ask:

- "Is the grain wheat?" (Yes)

- "Are you allergic to any other grains?" (No)

- "What is it in the wheat you are allergic to? Is it the bran?" (No)

- "Is it the gluten?" (No)

- "Is it the germ?" (Yes)

- "Do you have any other food allergies?" (No)

Foods and possible allergen agents:

Food	Allergy agents
Wheat	Bran, Gluten, Germ
Milk	Fats, Calcium, Lactose, Enzymes, additives
Chocolate	Caffeine, Fats, Pesticides, Cockroaches
Citrus Foods	Citric Acid, Bioflavonoids
Peanuts	Fats (use almond butter instead)

You can test a particular organ to see what the allergy is.

- "Are the allergies in your nose to something you are eating?" (Yes)

- "Is it milk?" (Yes)

- "Are there any other food allergies in your nose?" (No)

- "Are the allergies in your nose to something you are breathing also?" (Yes)

Testing breathing allergies

- "Are the allergies in your body to something you are breathing?" (Yes)

- "Is it pesticides?" (No)

- "Is it chemicals?" (Yes)

- "Is it perfumes?" (Yes)

- "Is it car exhaust?" (Yes)

- "Is it cigarette smoke?" (Yes)

- "Are there pollens you are allergic to?" (Yes)

- "Is it grasses?" (No)

- "Is it weeds?" (Yes)

- "Is it bushes?" (No)

- "Is it trees?" (Yes)

If you are a horticulturist, you can test for exactly WHICH trees, bushes, grasses, or trees.

When I find a lot of breathing allergies, I ask:

- "Are chemical allergies your most severe?" (Yes)

There are chemicals in nearly every thing you can think to test for except the pollens. Pesticides, perfumes, gas/diesel exhausts, cigarette smoke, and air pollutants all have chemicals of some kind in them.

Some people are more sensitive to chemicals than others. If that is the case, their body will react to many airborne allergens.

Every single person I test has an allergy to some degree or another to chemicals and/or perfumes. Some are severe; others are noticeable but not bothersome.

You know you are allergic to something if it smells very strong or stinky, takes your breath away, knocks your hat off, induces nausea, causes a headache, makes you cough, or makes you feel generally "sick" after smelling it.

It is impossible to control what other people wear, but it is possible to control your own environment. If a perfume or soap makes you sick, you don't have to use it; if a cleaning chemical makes you cough and choke while you are in the bathroom cleaning with it, pick a different cleaning chemical.

One person will put on a perfume she just loves. When she go out in public, someone she meets will fan his nose or mutter under his breath: "She sure doused herself in perfume today!"

Actually, the perfume wearer applied a small dab to her neck or wrist. It smelled good to her. The one who is allergic to it can't stand the smell or strength of it.

Testing for touch allergies

- "The rash on your skin, is it an allergic reaction to something you are eating?" (No)

- "Is it to something you are breathing?" (No)

- "Is it to something you are touching?" (Yes)

- "Is the allergy to chemicals?" (Yes)

- "Is the allergy to animal dander?" (No)

- "Is the allergy to laundry soap?" (Yes)

- "Is it the chemical in the soap?" (Yes)

It is possible to test for each individual product on the label if you want to isolate the exact chemical that is a problem. A chemist would have fun with this!

My sister works for a dentist. She had problems with her ears. We tested it to be an allergy to chemicals at work. She knew the names of the various dental and cleaning chemicals they used.

As she said the name of the product, I tested her on each one. We were able to isolate the three products that bothered her.

She had a weeks vacation from work, so I reset her body against those chemicals and it worked!

I did not know the product, but her energy did. Therefore, I could ask her energy and trust it would tell me what it knew about the products she was exposed to.

Several changes in the way we live have contributed to the increase in allergies. Following are a few of the main factors.

1. We are keeping our homes warmer and cooler without opening windows or doors when we need fresh outside air.

2. Foods are sprayed with pesticides and insecticides, then processed with preservatives to enhance shelf life. These products are not compatible with the live cell process.

3. Chemicals in the air from cars, factories, and spray products add to poor air quality.

4. Stress created by crowded living conditions overworks the immune system.

5. Generally speaking, most diets do not include enough fresh fruits, vegetables, whole grains, and nuts to keep the body functioning and healthy. A healthy person has less allergies.

6. Allergies seem to be more pronounced in mountainous regions due to increased plant and pollen life.

When inversions trap pollutants right next to the ground, those allergic to chemicals or other airborne allergens are forced to breathe them in heavier concentration than they would on a clear sunny day. These people really do feel better on sunny days than when it is cloudy or overcast. They may think they are "sun worshipers", when in reality, they are "chemical sensitive".

All of us have allergies at varying degrees of severity. It's good to know what they are.

Bio-Kinetic testing provides the guidelines to discover those allergies and then deal with them.

BACTERIA

Bacteria were first observed under a simple microscope by a Dutch naturalist named Anton van Leeuwenhoek. The source and purpose of bacteria was debated for years until 1860 when Louis Pasteur discovered that bacteria were the cause of many infectious diseases. Thus arose the train of thought that EVERY disease was caused by bacteria. Recent discoveries of viruses, parasites, yeast and allergic reactions have refuted this as fact.

Since the discovery of bacteria, many methods have been explored to develop immunity to bacteria-related illnesses. These include diseases such as typhoid fever, tetanus, tuberculosis, plague, syphilis, cholera, lockjaw, leprosy, and several forms of pneumonia, to mention a few.

Three Types of Bacteria

There are many types of bacteria. Three of the main groups are:

1. Those that live on dead animal and vegetable matter, decomposing it and returning it to mother earth to be used by future living plants. Bacteria that destroy dead material are vital to the life cycle.

2. Those that are parasitic, or co-exist with a living host. The parasitic-bacteria is usually absent from normal tissue, but it is found in the digestive tract where it is indispensable in normal intestinal functions.

3. Those bacteria that are disease producing. The pathogenic (or disease-producing bacteria) invade the body from outside and cause infection.

The bacterium in numbers 2 and 3 deal with personal physical health.

Remember the law of opposites. Yeast and bacteria occur naturally in the digestive tract and provide a healthy balance.

Things that can upset that delicate balance are improper diet, taking harmful products into the body, stress, angers and tension, chemicals, preservatives, antibiotics, etc.

The pathogenic bacteria invade body tissue and release a type of chemical or poison called toxins into the body fluids. The toxins released by one type of bacteria are different than the toxins released by another type.

Certain things produce chemicals that can control, if not destroy, bacteria. Among other things, these include vitamins, herbs, and antibiotics. Until recently, antibiotics have been more heavily favored as a bacteria control than either diet or herbs.

We are most familiar with the bacteria STREP. This is equated with rheumatic heart disease.

Lesser known but still a threat to the body is STAPH. This one is more popular in hospitals where it seems to flourish in nurseries and operating rooms.

Staph frequently exists on the skin and should reside on the outside. An untreated open wound will allow this to enter and invade local cells.

Here is an example of how Bio-Kinetic testing works hand in hand with medical science.

One of my clients brought her son to be tested. He had a sore toe that had bothered him for a couple of days.

It was red with a pus build up in the center. My testing revealed it to be staph.

I tested him for herbs and topical products but told the mother to watch the toe very carefully. If she saw any red streaks going up the foot, she should take him to a doctor immediately.

She decided to have it tested the next day because this news concerned her. The doctor looked at it and declared it to be gout. However, with further testing, it became obvious to her doctor that it was staph.

This put the young man in the hospital with IV's running antibiotics into his veins for a week.

This is the seriousness of a staph infection.

When my children get a cut or a hangnail, we put cayenne pepper on it along with a band-aid. This will draw out bacteria of any kind. Using preventive methods keep a staph from getting worse.

We were in the mountains one time on a family picnic. One of my boys stepped on a piece of broken glass in a stream. I happened to have cayenne with me. We put copious amounts on the cut and applied a band-aid. The bleeding stopped immediately and the cayenne promoted healing.

The next day he was walking on it without any pain, and it healed up without even a scar.

This is the beauty of herbs when battling bacteria or any type of injury or infection.

Certainly I would have taken my son to see a doctor had I seen the cut developing into a severe situation.

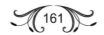

YEAST INFECTION

Friendly yeast is present in the digestive system. Yeast is capable of causing disease in an unhealthy individual. How ill someone becomes with a yeast infection will depend greatly on the strength of his immune system.

The occurrence of candida (or yeast) infection seems to parallel the arrival of antibiotics. This is what I have traced most yeast or candida to when I have tested for its source.

Antibiotics may have been used mainly during childhood, but it was enough to upset the delicate balance of the body so that years later there is still an ongoing battle with yeast or candidiasis.

The most common difficulty faced by sufferers of yeast is that there is no known way of testing for overgrown yeast. Since yeast occurs naturally in the system, it shows up as normal on tests. Guide-lines need to be established to determine what is normal and what is out of range.

The majority of medical doctors are not absolutely convinced that this is a legitimate medical illness.

Common symptoms of yeast infection include headache, memory loss, hyperactivity, irritability, fatigue, depression, kidney and urinary problems, stomach or digestive ailments, skin eruptions, vaginitis, sexual dysfunction, aching muscles, bones and joints, and other health complaints.

These can be symptoms of other diseases, too. This is where Bio-Kinetic testing is so valuable. Yeast cannot hide from the quick eye and hand of one who is alert to it.

Women are most prone to yeast. I hear all the time about vaginal irritation from yeast. However, men can also get a yeast infection. A man will feel the physical effects of yeast just like a woman.

The best cure I've seen (and the cheapest) for a vaginal yeast is raw garlic. A bulb of garlic contains several sections called cloves, ranging in size from small to large.

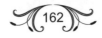

Peel the largest clove piece, score the inner skin slightly with a knife so the oils can be released, and then insert the clove vaginally at bedtime like a tampon. The next morning it usually is expelled into the toilet. If not, it can be retrieved with the index finger.

This is repeated every night until the irritation subsides.

Garlic releases its oils all night to counteract local yeast.

If a pregnant woman is infected with candida, her baby may be born with the infection. It shows up symptomatically as thrush, which is a white coating or spots on the tongue that look at first like curdled milk.

Thrush can spread and fill a baby's mouth. A nursing mother may pass yeast back and forth from her nipple to the baby's mouth.

Her baby will have a dry mouth, want to nurse more often, and may be extra fussy. A dry mouth is a sore mouth.

Yeast in the nipples is very painful. It will cause sore, dry, cracking nipples.

In a following section on testing for vitamins and herbs, I will talk about supplements that have been known to help relieve symptoms of a yeast infection.

Yeast Diet

Diet is important and should exclude the following: no bakers yeast, no refined sugars, no mushrooms or fungus foods, no wines or liquors, no fruits that are very sweet, high in fiber or have an edible skin. These fruits include apples, grapes, blueberries, strawberries, watermelon, and cantaloupe.

Stay away from corn products (anything with the word "corn" on it) and alcoholic beverages. Both seem to have the effect of feeding a yeast infection.

Citrus fruits are more acidic and are fine if you are not allergic to them.

A banana a day is usually tolerated since bananas are more easily digested by the body. However, several bananas may not be good. Test to see how many can be eaten without causing additional yeast problems.

Pineapple juice is a substitute for sugar. Pure, raw honey from a local bee man or blackstrap molasses are also good sugar substitutes.

There is some controversy over commercially produced sugar substitutes. Bio-Kinetic testing will determine if you can use sugar substitutes in the place of sugar. If not, you should consider one of the above-mentioned alternatives.

There is a handy and concise reference tool located in the appendix listing all the do's and don'ts for the yeast diet.

VIRUS

Have you ever tried to pinpoint the exact number of known viruses? Each year this seems to change as new and more dreaded viruses surface.

A few viral-related diseases are rabies, polio, yellow fever, measles, mumps, chicken pox, the herpes viruses, some forms of acute diarrhea, warts, hepatitis, the many different cold and flu viruses, respiratory virus, Epstein-Barr, etc.

Viruses are spread through people-to-people contact; by droplets coughed or sneezed into the air; from contact with contaminated feces or urine; or by biting insects.

Little can be done medically for viruses except to "go home, take two aspirin, and call me in the morning."

This phrase has been a disappointment to many, as well as a source of many puns leveled at the medical profession—all because of a virus!

On the other hand, herbs and vitamins have been known for years to have a profound effect on viral invasions.

There are those who have done research on vitamin C and provided information to substantiate that high doses of vitamin C have very beneficial effects on the immune system. The RIGHT kind of vitamin C for each individual is the best defense against a viral attack.

With Bio-Kinetic testing, you can determine whether your chemical make up allows you to use an over-the-counter vitamin C, or if you do better with one manufactured by and sold through health food stores.

Epstein-Barr Virus

This virus appears to be the most misunderstood of all the viruses. From the years of testing that I have done with my clients, I have come to one conclusion: this is occurring in plague proportion.

For this purpose, I am devoting as much time and attention to this virus as I can so you might become acquainted with it and its symptoms.

There seems to be a magical charm with this virus and the host body. I have tested people in their fifties and sixties who were born with the virus and have never known a day of feeling well.

One of my clients was in his late fifties. He had been born with the Epstein Barr Virus and had never remembered feeling healthy or energetic his whole life.

After following the program with me, within a month his health was better than he had ever known. He leaned towards me and said, "Well, Tisha, now I have my life back, I don't know how to act or what to do with myself!"

I recommended he go hiking, dancing, climbing a mountain, or taking his wife to all the exotic places he had only been able to dream about for years.

A long term illness will develop a habit of thinking you are ill. I suggested to my client that he change his way of thought as well as his lifestyle.

Invariably when a client gets over Epstein Barr, the response is, "Wow, is this how life is supposed to feel?"

Why does it stay around so long when most viruses can be overcome within a few days, or at the most a few weeks?

It apparently has the ability to confuse the immune system into thinking it belongs there or it wouldn't be around for so long. From what I have been able to detect, the virus invades a host cell, and when the cell reproduces, it also passes on the genetic DNA for Epstein-Barr. Thus, a new cell and a new virus agent are born.

I have never seen Epstein-Barr alone kill anyone, although many feel half-dead because it is so exhausting.

Over time, Epstein-Barr weakens the immune system. This allows other illnesses a better chance of invading and gaining strength because the T-cells are worn out in the continuing battle with the Epstein-Barr virus.

I compare it to sending out grown soldiers with armor and swords to begin the fight but, as the battle drags on, trained and skilled warriors give way to babes in diapers who become the major defenders.

From the testing I have done, I find Epstein Barr to be the main culprit in such diseases as the Chronic Fatigue Syndrome, Mononucleosis, hyperactivity, depressions, anxieties, intestinal complaints, headaches, along with complaints of malaise, aching and/or flu like symptoms so many people experience.

Become familiar with this virus. It has so many symptoms associated with it that I have decided to label it with a Dr. Jekyll, Mr. Hyde syndrome.

I have traced Epstein-Barr virus to three origins:

1. If a pregnant woman has this in her uterus, it can be passed on to her newborn. Her baby will be quite sickly. He will either be lethargic, or the exact opposite—very fussy and hyper. A baby that screams nonstop for 24 hours can unnerve even the most patient of parents.

2. Vaccinations contain the virus. The Epstein-Barr needs a host cell as a passport to your body. With the viruses used in immunizations, the Epstein-Barr virus has an instant host provided to transport it directly into your system. Many times I have heard the comment, "I got those shots, walked out of the office, and have never been the same" or "I got the flu shot and was sick with the flu all winter." It was really Epstein-Barr Virus.

    One family I worked with had a baby who received immunizations. Two weeks later he was in the hospital with viral pneumonia. He was given intravenous antibiotics. The end result of that was a raging yeast infection.

    When he was released, his mother brought him to see me. We were able to successfully rid his system of both the infections, and he was much healthier.

    Vaccinations have their place. As you read on, you will see that Bio-Kinetic testing waylays the illnesses or reasons for the immunizations.

    My children are learning about herbal usage and how to test themselves when an illness arises. I feel confident that they will be able to prevent many of the plagues and diseases that sweep the earth.

This is not the case with those who live in undernourished or poverty conditions. Under circumstances such as these, vaccinations are a valued option to saving lives.

3.   This virus spreads from one person to another like a common cold. Mononucleosis is called "the kissing disease" for an obvious reason. Mono is an indication that the Epstein-Barr virus exists in the body.

I tell my teenagers, "Bring that date in and let me test him/her before you kiss goodnight."

Their response? "Yea, right!"

One of my sons picked up Epstein-Barr from using a computer keyboard that an employee from a previous shift worked on. He didn't wash his hands before eating lunch. Lack of personal hygiene is a personal invitation to the Epstein-Barr virus. Another child got it when a fellow football player drank out of his water jug at practice. A daughter picked it up after a sleep over with a friend. I could hear her friend coughing during the night and sure enough, being confined to close quarters with an infected individual left my daughter wide open for the infection. The stories go on and on.

Epstein-Barr virus has many symptoms. It will manifest itself according to the body organ it is in at the time. It can be absolutely eradicated from your body with herbs and diet, only to re-enter under optimum conditions at some future time. Should you pick it up again, your symptoms may vary, because more than likely it will settle in a different organ.

Following are some of the symptoms possible when Epstein-Barr invades particular organs.

Bones. One client I worked with had been diagnosed with arthritis. Her bones ached constantly. A medical doctor suggested she take steroids and gold shots for it. After doing the Epstein-Barr cleansing, one month later she was washing walls, packing boxes, and moving to California—without a bit of pain. It was Epstein-Barr in her bones, not arthritis.

Brain. I have worked with high school students who were straight "A" students until they got Epstein-Barr in the brain, which caused their grades to plummet. After ridding the brain of the Epstein-Barr virus, their good grades returned. The only reason these students could do this is because they had developed effective study habits already. We make no claims that getting rid of Epstein-Barr will give you excellent grade reports, but that would be nice!!

Epstein-Barr in the brain causes a confusion of thought, headaches, inability to concentrate, loss of memory, and many classic symptoms of multiple sclerosis.

Ears, nose, or throat. When this virus settles in the head, it causes constant infections, congestion, sinusitis, cough, and mucous drainage. The end result for children is usually a medical procedure to place tubes in the ears. Lots of antibiotics may be used for constant ear, nose, and throat infections. Antibiotics are for bacteria, they do nothing for a virus, and only lead to a yeast overgrowth.

Heart. If Epstein-Barr settles for a period of time in the heart muscle, it may weaken the heart. Symptoms include heavy palpitations, skipping of beats, shooting pains, heaviness in the chest—all the typical symptoms of heart disease. Heart tissue that has been weakened by disease can be restored to normal. Genetic abnormalities do not fall under this category.

Liver and lymphatic system. Epstein-Barr virus in these organs causes definite symptoms of Chronic Fatigue, and Mononucleosis. The symptoms are extreme tiredness; falling asleep in a chair at the drop of a hat; lumps and swellings in various parts of the body because the lymph nodes are full of the virus; the liver will "ache" which feels very much like a gallbladder attack.

Stomach and large intestine. A person with Epstein-Barr in the stomach and/or large intestine feels nauseated; becomes a picky eater; develops pains in the stomach; has bowel problems such as diarrhea, abdominal cramps, constipation, or gas.

A 12-year-old boy I worked with had Epstein-Barr since birth. His mother said he had been a "spitty" baby who screamed with abdominal pain. She thought he had an extreme case of colic. As he grew up, he was a

finicky eater, which was very disconcerting to his mother. After working with me on an Epstein-Barr cleansing program for a couple of months, his mother called me and said, jokingly of course, "I almost wish he had it back! He is eating me out of house and home!!" They were obviously relieved to see him so healthy.

Nervous system. A nervous system full of Epstein-Barr causes symptoms of irritability; headaches; depression; anxiety; numbness or tingling down the arms and shoulders or legs and feet; fibromyalgia; bad dreams; sleeplessness; inability to sleep because the mind is going "100 miles an hour"; or waking up in the middle of the night unable to get back to sleep.

Kidneys or bladder. Epstein-Barr cause such things as bed-wetting; urinary urgency; urinary incontinency; low back ache; blood in the urine; and pain or pressure in the bladder. Those who have Epstein-Barr in the kidneys or bladder are no fun to travel with. They keep asking, "Are we there yet . . . I mean to the rest stop?"

Female sex organs. When Epstein-Barr harbors in the female sex organs, it will cause irregular periods; heavier bleeding, or less bleeding; extreme hormone changes that feel like constant PMS; severe menstrual cramps with the period; painful intercourse; miscarriages; and/or endometriosis if left unattended for many years. It has also been known to cause symptoms similar to those of a vaginal yeast infection with itching, burning, and irritations.

Male sex organs. Male sex organs infected with Epstein-Barr virus cause the prostate to swell and create pressure and pain with symptoms of prostatitis. These include getting up frequently at night to go to the bathroom; urinary urgency; urinary frequency; or inability to urinate. Epstein-Barr can also cause the testes to be inflamed, which contributes to painful sexual relations.

Other symptoms to watch for with this virus could include such things as skin rash, skin eruptions or lumps of any kind, aches, fever, chills, flu-like symptoms, dizziness, and muscle weakness.

Epstein-Barr virus goes through cycles where it will flare up or be considered active, then it will go into remission. When it is active the physical symptoms will vary depending on the organ or organs it infects at the time. After days,

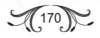

weeks, months or years of this, the immune system is then able to battle it into remission.

One of my clients had been bedridden for three years before she came to see me. It took her immune system that long to be able to battle the virus into remission.

When it goes into remission, it lies dormant in a particular organ or two before it flares up again days, weeks, months, or years later, depending on the strength of the immune system to keep it at bay.

Each time it flares up, another organ becomes the recipient of it's unleashed fury. After several episodes of this, many organs become involved, and the symptoms become more and more pronounced and severe.

The longer the person has had this virus, the more frequent the flare ups become and the longer the body will remain in a weakened condition.

It is like a roller-coaster ride of health.

Epstein-Barr Diet

It is important to eliminate certain foods.
- Fats because they plug up the liver, and the liver is a vital organ in fighting off the virus. Some foods high in fats are cheese, ice cream, chocolate, fatty icing, high-fat salad dressings, red meats (pork is a red meat), deep-fried foods like chips, french fries, donuts, pastries, shortening, butter, etc.

- Wines and liquors because they adversely affect the liver,

- Potatoes, tomatoes, green peppers, and eggplant. These foods seem to be a breeding ground for the virus. If you get rid of the breeding ground, you get rid of the virus a lot faster.

By spending a lot of time discussing Epstein-Barr does not mean we de-emphasize other viruses. Many cold, flu, respiratory, and childhood diseases hit us every year. Not every virus is Epstein-Barr.

Testing for a virus

- "Do you have a virus?" (Yes)

- "Is it Epstein-Barr?" (No)

- "Is it a cold virus?" (No)

- "Is it a flu virus?" (Yes)

- "Is it a respiratory virus?" (No)

Then you can test for vitamins and herbs to help assist the body in getting over that particular virus. These will follow in the section titled "Testing for Vitamins and Herbs."

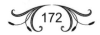

PARASITES

Funk and Wagnall's Encyclopedia describes parasites as:

> *"Any organism living on or in another living organism, and*
> *deriving part or all of its nutrients from the host without*
> *contributing anything to the host. In most cases, parasites damage*
> *or cause disease in the host." (Funk and Wagnalls New*
> *Encyclopedia, Volume 20, pg. 149.)*

Parasites are not met with much enthusiasm when they are tested as existing within the organs of a human being! One of the most amazing parasites is the tapeworm. It is transparent with a suction mouth that attaches to the wall of the small intestine. It can grow to incredible lengths and live for years in the intestine. It waits for food to come through so it can absorb it through the cells of its body. Basically it becomes a robber within the system, robbing you of vital nutrients.

Other types of parasites that are known to invade the human body are fluke worms, roundworms, pinworms, protozoa, amoeba, and parasitic bacteria.

Not too many children get through their childhood years without experiencing the itch and misery of pinworms. These are small white worms that are passed through animal feces into the dirt or carpets where little children sit and play.

Once inside the system this parasite can be a contributing factor to bed-wetting. The worms crawl to the rectum during the night to lay their eggs which causes a child to itch and scratch and toss and turn. This stimulates the bladder to empty.

Another common parasite is the roundworm. Roundworm eggs are generally passed from one host to another through food or unsanitary conditions. Once inside the body, the worm will settle in the large intestine waiting for food to pass from the small intestine where they gobble up nutrients intended for its host.

Few people who have traveled to other parts of the world come back without some kind of intestinal "souvenir." The diarrhea, stomach cramps, gas, and nausea that attend the amoeba or bacterial-type parasites is intense.

They are caused by microscopic parasites who find that the intestines are a nice warm place to multiply and divide—time and time again. This can go on for years.

I worked with a Viet Nam veteran who had been home 30+ years and had intensifying intestinal problems. Tests were run and tubes were "poked in every open orifice" (direct quote). He was given x-rays and asked to swallow all kinds of "interesting things." Nothing showed up. I tested him and found a host of parasites. After a month on parasite cleansing herbs, all his symptoms went away.

Some parasites crawl through the body and attack vital organs. They have been known to attack the liver, the heart, and even the brain.

It is rare, but there have been a couple of women I have tested who had parasites in the uterus.

One lady was pregnant. In about the third month of pregnancy her embryo just "magically disappeared." Her doctor told her it appeared to have been eaten up or something.

When I tested her, I found parasites in the uterus. We got her cleaned out, and later she was able to conceive and bear a healthy baby boy.

One of the obvious symptoms of intestinal parasites is a gurgling or rumbling stomach. People say, "I sit in church and feel so embarrassed because my stomach is louder than the preacher."

I tell them, "Those are just the 'little bugs' singing their praises but soon they will sing a different song as we escort them out of the human temple".

Parasites can be eliminated with herbs.

When someone has parasites, we do NOT do vitamins for two weeks while we do a parasite cleanse. I have found that vitamins simply serve to "fortify" the bugs.

After two weeks on an herbal cleanse, vitamins and minerals can be added as tested for.

CANCER

Cancer is viewed as a terrible illness that more than likely will result in death. Cancer is described as a rapid growth of abnormal cells. These cells have the ability to take over and invade surrounding tissue. Good evidence exists that cancer starts in a single cell that somehow goes "berserk" and does not respect the body's control mechanism of cell growth.

Cancer cells have the capability of spreading to other parts of the body. When this happens, we say the cancer has metastasized.

Under optimum conditions, healthy body cells manage to eat up or destroy the cancerous ones. One of the conditions that encourages this is fasting. During a fast, the body will feed on itself and destroy the old and defective cells first.

Other habits that help rid the body of cancer are a good diet, adequate rest, proper vitamins and herbal therapy, and a positive outlook on life.

The book of Job in the Holy Bible tells us the part mental attitude may play in the development of cancer.

> *"For the thing which I greatly feared is come upon me, and that which I was afraid of is come unto me." (Job 3:25.)*

Another good scripture is 2 Timothy 1:7

> *"God hath not given us the spirit of fear."*

Fresh fruits and vegetables are a great deterrent to cancerous growths. The American Cancer Society tells us that fresh broccoli and cabbage have cancer inhibiting properties. Others have worked successfully with wheat grass, vitamins, herbs, massage, mental healing suggestions, humor, chelation therapy, and living in stress-free, non-polluted conditions.

Cancer is best left to be diagnosed by health-care professionals. If there is ever a doubt about it, recommend the client go see a doctor for a complete medical check-up. Suggestion: Test herbs for virus and/or Essiac Formula on page 231 for help with cancer. If cancer is caught in the early stages, it is reversible.

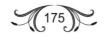

SEXUALLY TRANSMITTED DISEASES

There are several types of sexually transmitted diseases (STDs). The most familiar are syphilis, gonorrhea, AIDS, and herpes.

STDs show up as warts, parasites, virus, or bacteria. It is possible to have more than one STD at a time.

AIDS is probably the most feared of all the STDs. It is a virus. Some of the symptoms of AIDS are headache, fatigue, fever and chills, white tongue, intestinal distress, and eventual failure of other organs.

Syphilis is a bacteria that can be contracted through kissing someone who is infected or through sexual intercourse. In the early stages it may be manifest by a sore on the sex organs, a rash, or a sore throat. There may be redness and swelling around the rectum accompanied by a fever.

Gonorrhea is a bacteria and has no early symptoms. It can lie in the body cavity to be passed to the next sexual partner, and even passed on to babies. I had a client who adopted a baby. The baby had a pussy discharge from her vagina and rectum and had what the mother thought to be a diaper rash. Since this was her first baby, she had no idea this was not normal. The baby had been infected by her birth mother or father.

Gonorrhea causes painful intercourse and urination. If the male has pus coming from the penis, he probably has gonorrhea.

Herpes: There are several types of viral herpes. Herpes simplex shows up in the mouth, causing sores or cankers. This can be contacted from kissing someone who has the disease, or from sharing spoons or straws with an infected person.

Genital herpes is passed though sexual contact. Its symptoms include itching and irritation. The symptoms are very similar to a yeast infection. A herpes or Epstein-Barr virus can cause the same itching.

Other symptoms include a clear discharge from rash-like eruptions on the vaginal area or penis. It is possible to have a herpes flare up on the hands, nose, or any skin area, which looks like red weepy eczema. A newly-wed friend of mine noticed this on her husband's fingers. Later she broke out with a raging vaginal herpes infection.

Chlamydia is another STD that initially has no symptoms. It shows up later with a cheese-like discharge accompanied by itching and burning which is common also to yeast infection. Painful intercourse is present with this disease in both male and female. The male will experience a watery discharge from the ureter. Chlamydia in a female can predispose her to a tubular pregnancy.

Genital warts are very similar to warts on the skin. They tend to grow in clusters. They will show up anywhere around the openings to the sex organs or will grow inside the vaginal tract close to the uterine cervix.

Cervical dysplasia is abnormal tissue in the cervix and is a precancerous condition. The belief is that this is caused by the same virus that causes genital warts.

I worked with a client who had been married previously to a promiscuous husband. They had several children together when she divorced him and remarried. She had a hard time conceiving with her new husband. Bio-Kinetic testing revealed four sexually transmitted diseases, one of which was genital warts.

When she checked herself digitally, she could feel a cluster of warts on her cervix.

We tested and customized an herbal formula for her which took about two months to complete. At the end of the two months, she no longer felt the warts and within a few months she conceived and bore a healthy baby boy.

I worked with another woman who had been infected with four STDs for several years. She had many medical tests run because of the intense and constant itching, irritation and pain.

The tests generally revealed nothing except a yeast infection which she was treated for time and time again. She experienced a tubular pregnancy and after years of uterine problems finally had a hysterectomy.

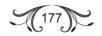

Before she consented to the hysterectomy, she came to me and we tried the herbs, but she had been infected for so long and with so many diseases they had damaged her uterus.

The pain and itching she endured for so many years was relieved with the hysterectomy. Surgery removed the diseases.

It's best to identify a sexually transmitted disease and get rid of it immediately. It's best yet to avoid getting infected in the first place.

Becoming informed, and then making wise choices would relieve much of the human suffering brought on by sexually transmitted diseases.

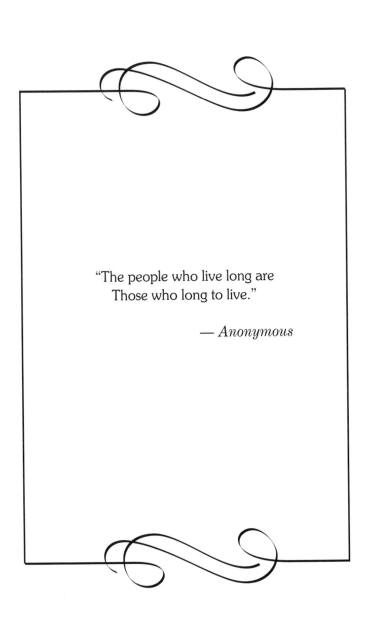

"The people who live long are
Those who long to live."

— *Anonymous*

CHAPTER 12

Testing on a Scale

Thanks to mathematical graphs and statistical charts, we have a basic understanding of scale ranges. The question is, "On a scale of 1–10, how do you rate?"

Bio-Kinetic testing utilizes this concept to detect degrees of physical weakness or strength.

On a scale of 1–10, 10 is always the highest, whether it is highest for the better or for the worst.

If we were testing a virus, for example, a "1" on the scale would be very minor but still detectable, whereas a "10" would be very high with all the symptoms. If you want to know the strength of any of your four rooms (physical, spiritual, emotional, mental), it is possible to measure 10+ + + and more if you wish, but "10" is a good stopping point. A "1" on the scale would be very low. A "10" would be perfect, healthy, or high. That is the ideal we all aim for.

I will say right here that the only ones I have tested who are a perfect "10" in all rooms are newborn babies. The rest of us have had a few more "knocks" during our existence in this physical world that can lower the numbers in those four rooms.

Testing yeast infection on a scale of 1–10:

- "On a scale of 1–10, with 10 being very high, how high is the yeast infection?"

"One?" (No)
"Two?" (no)

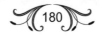

"Three?" (No)
"Four?" (No)
"Five?" (Yes)
"Six?" (No)

Swinging the feet for each number, it goes positive at the number five. This tells me the yeast is high enough to cause some symptoms but not terribly bad yet. Each organ can be tested the same way if you wish to detect what the number is in each organ.

This method can be used to measure severity of allergies, bacteria, virus infection, Epstein-Barr, cancer, nausea, headache, stress, or anything else.

Testing overall health on a scale of 1—10:

- "On a scale of 1—10, with 10 being very high, where is your overall physical health?"

"One?" (No)
"Two?" (No)
"Three?" (No)
"Four?" (Yes)
"Five?" (No)

Swinging the feet for each number, it goes positive on the number four. This means the physical health is only a four. Not very good when total good physical health is a 10.

This method can be used to measure the status of the four rooms: mental, emotional, physical and spiritual.

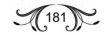

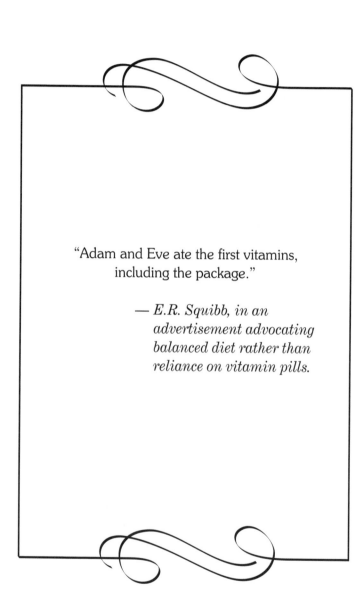

"Adam and Eve ate the first vitamins,
including the package."

— *E.R. Squibb, in an*
advertisement advocating
balanced diet rather than
reliance on vitamin pills.

CHAPTER 13

Vitamins

As a rule, a healthy body does not need a lot of vitamins on a continuing basis.

Children need a multiple vitamin when they are in a growth stage, and adults require a multiple vitamin mostly during times of illness, old age, severe stress, or pregnancy.

Some vitamins are fat soluble. This means that they will be stored in the body for a longer period of time. Because of this, fat-soluble vitamins are usually taken in low doses, every other day, or just two or three days of the week.

Fat soluble vitamins are A, D, E, FISH OILS, and LECITHIN.

Water-soluble vitamins include the B's and C's. These vitamins are used in amounts that the body needs at the time and then the rest are excreted from the body within hours. For this reason, water soluble vitamins need to be replaced every day.

Vitamin Information Table

VITAMIN	FOOD SOURCE	FUNCTION IN THE BODY
A	green and yellow veggie, egg yolk, carrots, fish liver oils	healthy bones, skin, eyes, sexual function, and reproduction
B1 (Thiamine)	whole grains, sprouts, beans, fresh green veggies, potatoes, carrots, brewers yeast	normal growth, promotes healthy appetite and heart; stimulates nerve impulses
B2 (Riboflavin)	wheat germ, eggs, seeds, green leafy veggies, brewer's yeast, peas, lima beans	skin, liver, eye health; fights anemia, stress, fatigue; prevents birth defects
B3 (Niacin)	fish, nuts, soybeans, poultry, meat, yeast, brewer's yeast	Heals skin and mouth sores; prevents stress, diarrhea, insomnia, abdominal pains, fatigue and irritability
B6 (Pyridoxine)	lean meat, fish, whole grains, soy, buckwheat flour, wheat germ, bananas, sunflower seeds, nuts	Cancer immunity; prevents diabetes, anemia, acne, asthma, depression, kidney stones, tooth decay, nausea & vomiting with pregnancy, menopause symptoms, menstrual symptoms
B12 (needs folic acid to be utilized)	yeast, wheat germ, milk, eggs, cheese	prevents anemia, nervous disorders, mental illness, promotes growth
Folic Acid	wheat bran, greens: beet, kale, spinach, asparagus, turnips	prevents problems in pregnancy; strengthens immunity; helps wounds heal
Biotin	eggs, whole grains, nuts, fish, wheat germ, brewer's yeast	prevents leg cramps; maintains skin, hair, nerves, sex glands, bone marrow

Choline	brewer's yeast, fish, soybeans, peanuts	liver, kidney, nerve function; builds immunity; strengthens heart
Inositol	brown rice, brewer's yeast, molasses	controls cholesterol; helps inhibit cancer; treats some nerve weakness
Pantothenic Acid	Brewer's yeast, peanuts, buckwheat, sunflower seeds	helps prevent fatigue, cramps, constipation, stress, arthritis; protects against radiation; builds immunity
PABA (Para-amino-benzoic acid)	eggs, molasses, brewer's yeast, wheat germ	helps form blood cells; prevents digestive disorders, depression, nervousness, sunburn, skin cancer
C	citrus fruit, rose hips, green peppers, broccoli, spinach, tomatoes, parsley, acerola cherry	necessary for healthy sex organs, adrenal gland, tissue repair, cartilage, skin, mental health; prevents cholesterol buildup, aging; helps heal wounds, anemia, arthritis, bruising, leg cramps, poisoning from toxic pollutants
D	cod & halibut liver oil, eggs, salmon, tuna, enriched milk, alfalfa, sunshine	healthy bones, nerve, heartbeat; regulates calcium absorption
E	green leafy veggies, whole grains, wheat germ, vegetable and safflower oil, peanuts	prevents aging, blood clots, cancer, wrinkles, skin ills, menopause symptoms, heart disease, varicose veins, resists pollution, builds fertility
F	flax seed oil	helps relieve prostate problems
K	green leafy veggies, egg yolk, tomatoes, wheat germ, soybeans, potatoes	assists with blood clotting; prevents bruising and hemorrhaging

MOST COMMONLY USED VITAMIN SUPPLEMENTS

B COMPLEX

Major infections like yeast and Epstein-Barr deplete the B vitamins. These particular vitamins are most beneficial to the nerves and the nervous system.

B complex (which is a combination of ALL the B's mixed together in a certain milligram amount) is the most effective way to take the B's. B Vitamins work better in combination.

Occasionally someone will test for an individual B if they have nerve trauma or are suffering with nausea during pregnancy or motion sickness of any kind.

The B vitamins are measured in milligrams or micrograms.

VITAMIN C

There are many different types of Vitamin C, including vitamin C with rose hips, vitamin C with bioflavonoids, ascorbic acid, citric acid, and ester-C. It is best to take vitamin C in individual doses several times a day instead of large doses all at once. The body can only utilize so much at a time.

If someone is allergic to citric acid or bioflavonoids, they need a vitamin C with rose hips only.

Vitamin C is measured in milligrams. Dosages start as low as 100 milligrams per tablet and go up in graduated amounts to over 2000 mg per tablet. Some are buffered, some are time released, some are chewable, and some are in crystal form that can be mixed with water or juice.

Vitamin C is water soluble, and the body will expel any amount it does not use. Vitamin C needs to be replaced every day.

Vitamin C can be given in large dosages (if you have tested for the type that is compatible), even up to 1000 mg/hr, the first day or two of an infection. Diarrhea is an indication that vitamin C is cleaning out the infection.

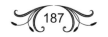

When someone is sick, if possible, they should be tested every day for vitamin needs. Individual physical requirements will change rapidly during illness.

Vitamin C is a key factor in healthy body cells.

VITAMIN E

Vitamin E plays a big role in immunity. It assists in the production of lymphocytes and antibodies. It has long been heralded as the "sex" vitamin, for it does fortify sexual function. Mixed with a cream base to be rubbed on the face and body, it can relieve wrinkling and scarring. The heart benefits from vitamin E, as does skin and liver stability. It is beneficial in combating the effects of pollutants and radiation.

Vitamin E comes in different strengths. It is fat soluble and CAN build up in the system if taken in large amounts. It strengthens the heart, but may contribute to heart problems if there is an overdose.

Vitamin E comes in IU's (international units.) It can be found as low as 100 IU's per capsule and as high as 1000 IU's.

Individual testing is important to see which brand, strength and type of vitamin E—if any—is needed.

LECITHIN

Lecithin is a brain food. It has the effect of strengthening the mental processes.

Human milk is rich in lecithin, while cow's milk is lacking in it. It is good to breast-feed babies as long as a mother is able.

Lecithin is fat soluble and stays in the system longer than water-soluble vitamins. It is high in choline and is a natural emulsifier of fats, which makes it helpful in fighting cholesterol build up.

Lecithin comes in strengths of up to 1200 mg and is available in capsules or in granules. In most cases, lecithin tests to be taken for two or three days out of the week instead of on a daily basis. It's important to test and see if lecithin is really needed and in which strength.

MULTIPLE VITAMINS

There are many brands of multiple vitamins on the market. Some people test well for generic brands, while others need the fruit and/or vegetable base.

A multiple vitamin eliminates the need for several individual vitamins.

A child in a growth spurt (a growth spurt usually lasts anywhere from 4-6 weeks), older citizens, a woman having her menstrual cycle, or is pregnant, or anyone suffering from some kind of a persistent illness are most likely to test positive for a multiple vitamin.

There are not a lot of C's or B's in a multiple vitamin, so they may have to be tested for and taken separate.

Multiple vitamins come with and without iron. Since some individuals have an intolerance to iron, always test to see if an iron additive would be the best.

VITAMINS A & D

These two vitamins are fat soluble. If the diet includes sea food regularly, then there should be adequate intake of these.

Test to see if they should be taken every day or just a couple of days out of the week.

TESTING FOR VITAMINS

Suggested order in which to test for vitamins:

- Multiple vitamin (with or without iron)

- B Vitamins (Complex? 50 or 100 mg.? Individual B?)

- Vitamin C (with rose hips, with citric acid, with Bioflavonoids, chewable, buffered, crystal, timed-released? Mg. Strength?)

- Vitamin A D E K (Circle the ones your client tests for.)

- Lecithin (Granules, capsules? Strength?)

With the hands in position for testing, use the same method used in testing for body parts.

Here are some things to consider when testing for vitamins:

1. Do you need vitamins?

2. What strength of the supplement?

3. How many of that particular vitamin do you need in a day?

4. What time of day would be best to take it?

5. How long can you stay on this vitamin?

- "Do you need vitamins?" (Yes)

- "Do you need a multiple vitamin?" (Yes)

- "Do you need a multiple with iron?" (Yes)

- "How many of the multiple vitamin do you need?"

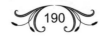
Testing for amounts

At this point, I will describe how to test for certain strengths of vitamins.

Swing the feet each time as you count by 1's, 5's, 100's, or 1000's according to milligram strength or number of tablets.

- "Do you need one?" (Yes)

- "Do you need two?" (No)

- "Do you want to take it in the morning?" (Yes)

- "Do you want to take it at night?" (No)

- "Do you need this every day for a long time?" (No)

- "Do you need this every day for a week?" (Yes)

- "In addition to the multiple, do you need a B vitamin?" (Yes)

- "Do you need a B50?" (Yes)

- "Do you need a B100?" (No)

- "How many of the B50 do you need a day? One?" (No)

- "Do you need two?" (Yes)

- "Do you need three?" (No)

- "Do you need one in the morning and one at noon?" (Yes)

The B complex gives energy, so it would be better to take them before 4:00 p.m.

- "Along with the multiple and the B complex, do you need a vitamin C?" (Yes)

- `"What kind of vitamin C is best for you? (Swing the feet for each kind of vitamin C you can think of) Do you need _____,(no) or _____,(No) or _____ (no) or _____?" (Yes)

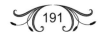

- "What strength of _____ do you want? 500 mg?" (Yes)

- "Do you want one?" (No)

- "Do you want two?" (Yes)

- "Do you want three?" (No)

The answer would be two. Both one and three say "no." This is a way of verifying the answer to keep going until you get a "No." The last number that tested "Yes" is the answer.

- "Do you want them both at once?" (No)

- "Do you want one in the morning and one at night?" (Yes)

- "Along with the multiple, the B vitamins, and the vitamin C, do you need any of the fat soluble vitamins?" (No)

If the answer is "Yes" then you would test each one of the fat soluble vitamins to see which one and which strength was needed.

- "Do you need Lecithin along with all the other things you just tested for?" (No)

The length of time to take a supplement can be accurate only to a degree. No one can see the future but God. We do not foresee stress, accident, trauma, or illness. If that should arise, then supplement needs will change.

This is one of the benefits of Bio-Kinetic testing. As life changes and circumstances are different, you can adjust daily supplements to meet your immediate need.

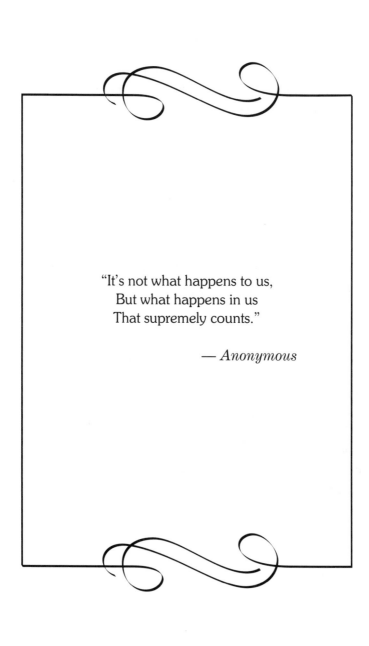

"It's not what happens to us,
But what happens in us
That supremely counts."

— *Anonymous*

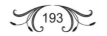

CHAPTER 14

Minerals

Minerals are nutrients essential to life. We would not be able to function without them. Minerals are found in the composition of teeth, bones, tissue, blood, muscle, and nerve cells.

Minerals run the electrical currents of the body. A proper ratio of minerals and vitamins is important for good health.

Minerals are found in the earth, and are absorbed into plant tissue from the ground where they are grown. Herbs are a rich source of minerals, as are organically grown fresh fruits, vegetables, whole grains, nuts, and seeds. Many of our soils today are lacking adequate mineral replacement. For this reason, mineral supplementation is vital to good health.

Minerals can also be deep mined or gathered from lake beds and oceans.

Minerals come in many forms. They can be taken individually or in combinations. Multivitamins will often be mixed with multiple minerals, or separated into vitamin combinations without minerals. Minerals are sold on the market in tablets, capsules, liquid, and powder form.

Some minerals are called essential minerals and are needed in larger amounts than trace minerals. Examples of essential minerals are calcium, magnesium, sodium, potassium, and phosphorus.

Some of the trace minerals include zinc, iron, copper, iodine, chloride, sulphate, boron, manganese, lithium, chromium, selenium, germanium, carbonate, bromide, fluoride, nitrogen, rubidium, scandium, nickel, strontium, cobalt, copper, tin, gold, silver, dysprosium, etc.

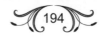

CALCIUM

In the 1960s, it was theorized that the "little old lady who had fallen and broken her hip had initial bone problems that caused her to bones to break." With today's knowledge, this has been verified. Studies done on osteoporosis show that bone mass thins, making it hard for the bones to sustain body weight. Therefore, the hip gives out and the person falls, breaking a hip.

Calcium is a major mineral that contributes to strong bones, teeth, and body strength. It helps coagulate the blood, and regulate the nerves, muscles, and heartbeat.

Calcium from a dairy source is not always digested or utilized. A strong indication from the testing I have done is that an individual who is allergic to the calcium in milk will have more of a tendency to bone weaknesses, IF milk has been his primary source of calcium. Some people absorb calcium from dairy, while others benefit from a plant or mineral source of calcium.

All the advertizing on earth will not convince me that everyone should drink milk to get "strong bones and teeth." Let's consider individual allergies and chemical make-up in deciding which calcium is best.

Calcium comes in chewable tablets, liquid, or solid-pressed tablets for easy swallowing.

Calcium supplements will likely contain vitamin D and/or magnesium to aid in it's absorption.

ZINC

Zinc is good for healing, for mental and physical development, and for cell production. Zinc and potassium have proven very helpful in easing skin problems. Teenagers would be wise to consider these before taking antibiotics for their "zits."

Zinc is important in the function of the immune system. The male reproductive organs especially benefit from zinc which has a positive effect on the prostate.

POTASSIUM

Along with sodium, this mineral is vital for the proper function of the sodium/potassium pump at the cell level. These two also control the water balance within the body. Potassium helps send messages along the nervous system and is an important factor in controlling the heart function. Excessive sugar, stress, salt, and alcohol destroy potassium.

IODINE

Iodine aids in proper function and restoration of the thyroid gland. Those who live inland away from fresh sea foods tend to have more thyroid malfunction. Sea foods are rich in kelp. Kelp is high in natural iodine.

CHROMIUM

Chromium plays a big role in metabolizing the glucose in the body and in helping with the production of insulin.

SELENIUM

This mineral works closely with vitamin E in fighting pollution and rebuilding healthy cells. It is a key factor in increasing immunity. It help in tissue elasticity.

Selenium is found in higher amounts in the pancreas, pituitary gland, and the liver. Supplementation with selenium can strengthen the immune system.

IRON

Iron comes in many types: ferrous gluconate, ferrous sulfate, chelated iron, iron and molasses, organic iron, iron in herbal bases, and so on. These are all basically iron, only in different forms. Lack of iron causes loss of energy, weakness and anemia. Too much iron can cause iron toxicity. Individuals should be tested for the correct type and amount of iron. Iron should be taken with food to make it less irritating to the stomach.

Seventy-five percent of the body's iron is in the blood. The rest is stored in the bone marrow, liver, spleen, and intestinal wall.

Most women test to need iron with their monthly cycle. Iron is lost with the loss of blood no matter what the cause may be. Iron supplementation begins the first day of the period and is used for about a week each month.

COPPER

An essential mineral involved in the storage and release of iron.

MAGNESIUM

Magnesium is important for the proper absorption of calcium allowed into the tissue. Calcium contracts the muscles; magnesium relaxes them. So, calcium and magnesium levels should be in the proper mix. Calcium supplements usually contain magnesium.

A lack of magnesium is believed to contribute to some heart ailments. Magnesium deficiencies may also contribute to calcified kidney stones, nervousness (Including PMS) and a nervous tick.

MANGANESE

This mineral is known to help control some forms of diabetes. It is also used to reduce high levels of copper in people with some forms of mental illness. It is important for reproductive function. Manganese deficiencies are linked with paralysis, deafness, dizziness, and ringing in the ears.

Manganese is helpful for mental clarity.

PHOSPHORUS

Calcium needs phosphorus to help form bone tissue. Most calcium supplements contain phosphorus.

Herbs are a natural source of vitamins and minerals. If you are using herbs, chances are you may not need additional vitamin or mineral supplementation.

Questions to ask about minerals:

- "Do you need additional minerals with the other products you are taking?"

- "Do you need a mix (or multiple) mineral?"

- "Do you need individual minerals?"

- "How many do you need a day?"

- "What time of day are they best taken?"

Testing for minerals:

- "Do you need minerals along with the other things you are taking?" (Yes)

- "Do you need a multiple mineral?" (Yes)

- "Do you need the mineral in tablets?" (No)

- "Do you need the mineral in liquid form?" (Yes)

- "How much of the mineral do you need?"

Testing for drops or ounces:

If the mineral is concentrated and is purchased in a container of eight ounces or less, then you would test for DROPS. If the container is larger than or exceeds ten ounces, then you would test to see how many ounces, half ounces or quarter ounces would be needed.

Ask these questions:

- "Do you need 5 drops/day?" (No)

Continue counting and swinging the feet for each drop until you get the correct number.

- "Do you need 15 drops?" (Yes)

- "Do you need 16 drops?" (No)

The same would be done with ounces. Start with one-half an ounce, then one ounce, then one and one half ounces , etc. until the right number is reached.

Testing for minerals in tablets:

- "Do you need a multiple mineral?" (Yes)

- "Do you want it in capsules?" (Yes)

- "How many capsules a day do you need? One?" (No)

- "Two?" (Yes)

- "Three?" (No)

- "Do you want them both at once?" (No)

- "Do you want one in the morning and one at night?" (Yes)

Testing for individual minerals:

- "Along with the vitamins, minerals and herbs you tested for, do you need an individual mineral?" (Yes)

At this point, you could test each individual mineral or, if you know the organ it would benefit, you could test the mineral best for that organ.

- "Is this mineral for you pancreas?" (Yes)

- "Do you need additional chromium?" (Yes)

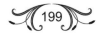

- "Do you need another individual mineral too?" (No)

- "How many chromium do you need? One?" (Yes)

- "Two?" (No)

- "Do you want chromium in the morning?" (No)

- "Do you want it at night?" (Yes)

Some minerals are not available in individual doses. Most of the minerals and amino acids are found in combination.

Here is a list to test from of a few of the minerals that are sold separate.

Multiple mineral	Chromium	Iron
Calcium	Selenium	Kelp
Zinc	Magnesium	Phosphorus
Potassium	Manganese	Other

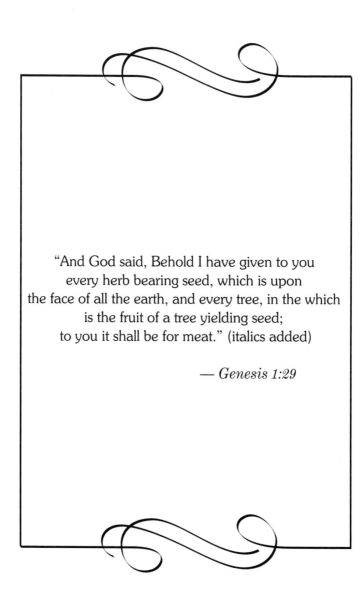

"And God said, Behold I have given to you
every herb bearing seed, which is upon
the face of all the earth, and every tree, in the which
is the fruit of a tree yielding seed;
to you it shall be for meat." (italics added)

— *Genesis 1:29*

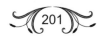

CHAPTER 15

Herbs

No claims are made here about the use of healing with herbs. For health problems, always seek the help and advice of a physician. Herbs should be used with judgement and skill.

The use of herbs is a fascinating and on going study. It becomes a life-time interest. As herbs are tested for and used, they get to be like old friends, both comfortable and welcome.

Herbs exist on every continent. Some can only be grown in a particular climate.

Having pondered this over the years, I think it is quite a wonder of the Creation that herbs were provided for people in every area of the earth. Think about how helpful this must have been before the advent of modern transportation. In this day and age, we can have an herb in our kitchen from the far reaches of Siberia or the rain forests of South America. This has not always been possible.

The modern herbalist has many more herbs at his command. Some herbs do much the same thing. Considering individual sensitivities, it is good that we have more herbs to choose from. When one herb is not tolerated, another herb can be used in it's place for the same symptom but without the side effects.

**NOTE: When testing for vitamins and especially herbs, be sure you find out if the individual is taking any prescription medicine!

MANY MEDICINES ARE NOT COMPATIBLE WITH CERTAIN VITAMINS OR HERBS.

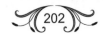

IF AN HERB DOES THE SAME THING AS THE MEDICINE, IT PROBABLY WILL NOT TEST TO BE TAKEN AT THE SAME TIME. An example: Heart medicine and herbs that strengthen the heart; Antidepressants and herbs for the nervous system; Diuretics and herbs for the urinary tract; Antibiotics and herbs that increase immunity.

Always test and ask the question: "Can this herb be taken with the medicine you are on?"

I was working with an individual whose parents came with him for testing. His mother asked me questions about using hawthorn for the heart. I recommended it's properties for heart weaknesses, but cautioned her about not taking it with any prescription heart medicine. She had given hawthorn to her husband who was already using a heart medication. When she gave him hawthorn he experienced dizziness and nausea.

This is a good example of the value of Bio-Kinetic testing. Had she known how to test, she would not have used hawthorn in connection with the medicine for she would have gotten a negative response through the INDICATORS.

RECOMMENDATION: Take Sunday off all supplementation (including vitamins, minerals, and herbs). Some herbs need two days' rest. Test and see how many days per week your body needs to rest from the health program you test for.

A day off of anything gives the body a chance to balance out on it's own.

If you are very ill or pregnant or having a monthly cycle, then the supplementation may need to continue even on Sunday.

The purpose of this book is not to educate you on herbs. The purpose is to teach you how to TEST for the herbs. For a more thorough study of herbs, consult other books on herbal usage. Herbs do come with cautions in combination with other products or during pregnancy. As always, becoming informed and knowledgeable about a subject gives you more confidence and power in your testing skill.

You will notice that some of the herbs are mentioned as being recommended for a 72 hour kit or invaluable in home usage. These are herbs I have found to be very useful in our family. You may find others that you feel more

comfortable with. As you begin working with herbs, you will find that every herbalist has their "favorite" herbs.

If an herb smells good or tastes good to you, you more than likely need that herb. To another person it will stink or be overpowering. It's likely his body has no need for that herb.

I had a female client who gave her husband a drink of Chamomile tea. She loved it and thought he would, too. He wrinkled his nose at the remembrance of the taste! Chamomile is more of a female hormone herb.

There are many books available about the use of herbs. You can read about everything from raising your own herb garden, to harvesting, drying, making tinctures, making poultices, arranging, gardening with, and medicinal usages. There are many great herb books available on any subject you wish to study. You will find them in your library or local health food store.

People ask me what books I recommend. I say, "It depends on your interest in herbs. Thumb through a book and if it appeals to you, that is the book you would learn something from."

I am going to give a brief explanation about some of the herbs I use the most. This is just a skeleton list of the many herbs available.

HOW TO BUY HERBS.

Herbs can be purchased in herbal capsules that have been filled and packed by an herbal company. Or, you can buy herbs in bulk packages from which you will make a tea or fill your own capsules. Herbs can also be purchased in liquid form.

Herbs come in cut, or powdered form. The cut herbs are used more for teas, whereas the powdered herbs can be put in gelatin capsules and swallowed. The teas and the liquid herbs are recommended for individuals who have a difficult time with swallowing. This could include small children or individuals with esophageal or abdominal complaints.

The gelatin capsules used for filling herbal capsules come in two sizes. "O" (pronounced "ott") and "OO" (pronounced "double ott"). "O" is the smallest, "OO" is larger.

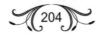

To fill the capsules, pull the two sections apart, fill both sides of the capsule with the herbal powder, put the sections back together and swallow the herbal-filled capsule.

Or, there are machines available that allow you to manually place the two halves of the capsule in small holes that hold the capsule in place. You fill the capsule halves with the powdered herb, fit the two sides of the capsule filling machine together, press firmly and the capsules snap together.

All the things you need for making your own capsules are available at health food stores.

COMMON HERBS:

ALFALFA: Builds blood and energy. Also very effective against the ravages of arthritis and bone disease. Very high in vitamins and minerals. Good for pituitary, liver and blood.

ANGELICA: Clean and strengthen uterus; relieves symptoms of endometriosis.

ASTRAGALUS: Boosts the immune system. Strengthens adrenal, kidney and lung function.

BARBERRY: Works in heart to decrease blood pressure. Strengthens lungs. Intestinal cleanser.

BAYBERRY: Helps with several female complaints. Good for cankers and sore throats. Cleans mucous out of the body.

BLACK COHOSH: Natural estrogen. Works on the heart, lungs, nerves, blood pressure and cholesterol.

BLACK WALNUT: Parasite cleansing. Helps relieve female disorders, sores in the mouth, throat and intestines.

BLADDERWRACK: Strengthens the thyroid. Used in weight maintenance formulas.

BLESSED THISTLE: Balances female hormones. Increases milk supply in nursing mothers. Works on circulation and lungs.

BLUE COHOSH: Used in childbirth. Relieves female complaints. Strengthens nervous system. Increases blood pressure.

BLUE VERVAIN: Aids female complaints. Works on colds and flu. Relieves nervousness and headaches. Removes mucous from the body.

BORAGE: Strengthens lungs and heart. Relieves skin problems that include ringworm, scabies, and insect bites. Relieves depression and mental anxieties.

BUCHU LEAVES: Works on endocrine system and is very effective in urinary, sex organ, and pancreatic weaknesses.

BUCKTHORN: Bowels and intestinal regulation. Expels worms.

BURDOCK: Excellent blood purifier. Used against STDs. Skin cleanser. Effective in kidney, urinary, liver and gallbladder problems. Strengthens bones and immunity.

BUTCHERS BROOM: Helps bones. Used in circulation disorders. Urinary and kidney cleanser.

CAPRYLLIC ACID: Not a true herb. Yeast fighter. Use this for two weeks only. Always take with food. After a few days break, it can be used again for the length of time tested for.

CAROB: Rich in vitamins and minerals. Great substitute for chocolate.

CASCARA SAGRADA: Aids in cleansing the intestines and bowels. Used as a natural, non-habit-forming laxative. Good for gall stones and liver cleansing.

CATSCLAW: Strengthens the immune, digestive, and bowel systems. Antioxidant. Used against arthritis, gastritis, tumors, female hormonal imbalances, cancer, virus infections, STDs, yeast and blood diseases

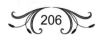

CATNIP: Colic relief. Works in fever and flu complaints. Relieve symptoms of chicken pox. Stress relief.

CELERY SEED: Decreases blood pressure. Helps bones and liver.

CAYENNE PEPPER or CAPSICUM: Cayenne should be planted in every yard or grown in a flower pot in every home. This is a universally known healing herb for many internal and external body ailments.

Cayenne is used for cuts; sore throats (1/4 tsp. Per 1/4 cup water); flu; aches and chills; heart and circulation; shock; combines with garlic for parasite cleansing; clears lungs, bronchial and sinuses; nosebleeds; infections of any kind; chills; endocrine system strengthener; urinary tract cleanser; ulcers; intestinal complaints; energy; and warming. Sprinkle in shoes if you live in cold climates. Cayenne is an herb that has been used in herbal formulas since the earliest civilizations.

CENTAUREA: Increase milk supply in nursing mothers.

CHAMOMILE OR CAMOMILE: Touch of female hormone. Soothing to nerves and intestines to promote restful sleep. Relieves headache and complaints associated with drug withdrawal. Effective pain relief in muscles and bones.

From our childhood memories comes the story about Peter Rabbit who ventured into Mr. MacGregor's garden. Peter had been warned by his mother not to go there for his father had recently lost his life in the garden. Adventuresome Peter disobeyed and after being discovered, chased by Mr. MacGregor, losing his new shoes and jacket, he arrived home in quite an upset state.

His mother put him to bed with chamomile tea while his sisters and mother enjoyed blueberry pie.

Chamomile is settling to the stomach and calming to the nerves.

CHAPARRAL: Systemic cleanser effective against radiation and formation of cancer cells. Good for skin, bones, kidney, lungs, liver.

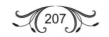

CHICKWEED: Cleanses and strengthens lungs and bronchi. Helps cleanse intestines, skin, tumor disorders and blood. Dissolves fat. Used in weight maintenance.

CLEAVERS: Kidney and bladder complaints. Cleanses blood and liver. Good for skin and childhood disease symptoms. Effective against STDs.

CLOVES: Used with parasite-cleansing herbs. Rids the system of parasite eggs. Useful against intestinal gas.

COMFREY: A blood cleanser. Very high in vitamin and mineral nutrients. The roots reach deep in the ground to absorb more nutrients than most herbs. Effective in skin, bone, muscle, lung, bronchial and intestinal complaints. Yeast fighter. Known to work on herpes, kidneys, and in poultices for sprains and bone trauma.

CORN SILK: Kidneys and urinary weaknesses. Natural diuretic.

CRANBERRY: Flushes kidney, ureter, bladder.

DAMIANA: Balances female hormones and is effective against hot flashes. Sex stimulant.

DANDELION: Builds blood and is rich in vitamins and minerals. Works on skin, bone, kidney and endocrine disorders. May help prevent cancer, age spots and anemia.

DULSE: Strengthens thyroid and other endocrine glands.

DONG QUAI: Female hormone problems especially those related to menopause. Used in childbirth. Opens circulation. Dissolves blood clots.

ECHINACEA: This herb cleanses the lymphatic system and supports the immune system. It is used with infections of the skin, blood, throat, as well as lymph system.

ELDERBERRY: Effective against viruses of all kinds, including STDs; treats the respiratory tract and throat.

EUCALYPTUS: Used for fevers, lungs, throat, sinus and respiratory problems. One teaspoon of the oil in one-half pint water, rubbed into the skin, is an excellent insect repellent. Watch for individual allergies to this herb.

EVENING PRIMROSE: Used in weight loss. Balances female hormone disorders. Used in bone complaints and skin disorders.

EYEBRIGHT: As the name suggests, it strengthens vision and can be used as an eye wash in cases of inflammation.

FALSE UNICORN: Used for female complaints associated with ovulation. Use small amounts only.

FENNEL: Intestinal gas and cramping. Relieves colic in babies. Increases milk production in nursing mothers. Works on kidneys, spleen, lungs, and bones. Removes radiation.

FENUGREEK: Great lung and bronchial cleanser. Works on intestinal gas, headache, and sore throat. Reduces fevers and cholesterol. Helps vision.

FEVERFEW: Pain relief in headaches, bones viruses and fever. Strengthens lungs and uterus.

FLAXSEED: Bones, nails, and teeth strengthener. Relieves constipation. Helps both male and female sex organ complaints. Especially good for the prostate.

GARLIC: Another wonderful herb that everyone should learn to use and accept. Garlic has been nicknamed the Russian antibiotic; it is anti-bacterial. Garlic is effective against yeast, bacteria, cancer and virus. It rids the system of parasites when used raw. Clears the skin and dissolves tumors. Very good for the heart, circulation, liver, lungs, ears, nose, throat and bronchi.

There is nothing like garlic and onion to build you up physically, and tear you down socially.

GENTIAN: Good for intestinal complaints, circulation, liver, spleen, and bones. Decreases fever.

GINGER: Works on lungs, kidneys, and bowels. Settles the intestines and helps in morning sickness and motion sickness. Used in bath water to ease aching muscles and remove toxins. It induces perspiration and clears the sinus and body of mucous. Effective against menstrual cramps and hot flashes.

GINKGO BILOBA: Memory and brain function. Good for kidney, circulation, and lung.

GINSENG: Connected with longevity. Helps in nerves, hormone balance, endurance, prostate, colds, lung function, immune system support, drug withdrawal, appetite stimulant, blood pressure, and endocrine gland support.

GOLDENSEAL: A very powerful healing herb used against infection, indigestion, flu, constipation, cankers, open skin sores, skin disease, urinary and bowel cleansing, ulcers, throat and gums, removes mucous. Strengthens function of the heart, lungs, liver, pancreas, sex organs, kidneys, blood and nerves.

Not to be used with low blood sugar. Used too long, goldenseal can promote yeast overgrowth just like an antibiotic.

GOTU KOLA: A great overall tonic for mental fatigue, senility, high blood pressure, and is reported to slow down the aging process. Increases energy and sex drive. Used in bone, urinary, nervous, STD, and mental disorders. Good for heart and liver function. Removes excess fluid.

GRAVEL ROOT: Cleanses the kidney, bladder, and gallbladder. Flushes calcifications.

GUARANA: Increases activity of endocrine system. Stimulant. Helps brain.

HAWTHORN: Valued as a heart tonic. Promising results have been reported in connection with a variety of heart ailments, including angina pectoris, high cholesterol and abnormal heart action. It is also believed to lessen the effects of hardening of the arteries. It has been used to treat arthritis, emotional stress, and nervous conditions.

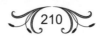

HOPS: Relieves nervous tension, acts as a sleep aid, and tones up the liver. Helps in alcohol withdrawal. Relieves symptoms of toothache, ulcers, pain, and cramps. Helps against gonorrhea.

HOREHOUND: Used to relieve coughs, colds, strengthens lungs, expel worms and afterbirth. A laxative in large doses.

HORSETAIL/SHAVEGRASS: Rich in silica this herb is good for bones, hair, skin, and nails. Cleanses kidneys and kidney stones. Good for eye, ear, nose, and throat complaints.

HUCKLEBERRY: Diabetes and insulin regulation. Useful in urinary problems.

HYDRANGEA: Works to remove kidney stones. Strengthens the urinary tract. Lessens the pain of arthritis and paralysis.

HYSSOP: Hyssop has been used in chest diseases and coughs, colds, hoarseness, fevers, and sore throats. It removes mucous and tumors from the body. Biblically it was used for cleaning sacred places.

ICELAND MOSS: Used in weight-maintenance programs. Effective against colds. Tones the body.

IRISH MOSS: Supports the thyroid and cleanses the body of fevers. Used in weight-maintenance programs.

JOJOBA: Healthy hair, skin, and scalp. Good against skin disorders like psoriasis and eczema.

JUNIPER BERRIES: Effective against diabetes, urinary and kidney weakness, bed-wetting, and yeast problems.

KAVA KAVA: Controls pain and cramps. Calms nerves.

KELP: Regulates the thyroid and pituitary glands. Good for healthy hair, skin, and nails. Removes the effect of radiation. Strengthens the nerves, brain, and spinal column. Strengthens sex glands.

LADY SLIPPER: Nerves and sleeplessness.

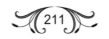

LICORICE ROOT: Good for hypoglycemia. It is a natural cortisone and helps with hormone balance. Licorice is a sex stimulant and is effective in balancing out monthly cycles that bring emotional swings and cravings. Strengthens the heart and circulation. Clears coughs and colds. Strengthens the voice. Is good against stress and intestinal disturbances.

LOBELIA: One of the stronger herbal relaxants known. Clears mucous out of the head, lungs, bronchi, and body so the body can heal. Effective against colds, headaches, rapid heartbeat, nerve and pain complaints, teething, and muscle spasms. Useful for cramping in any muscle. Reduces inflammation and fever and relieves symptoms of most contagious diseases. Combine with garlic and olive oil for ear infections.

MALE FERN: Eliminates worms from the intestinal tract.

MARJORAM: A sweet-tasting herb used with vegetables, turkey, and eggs. Dried leaves can be sprinkled on whole wheat bread and broiled slightly for a flavorful herb toast. Marjoram is used for headache and nervous complaints.

MARSHMALLOW: Effective against kidney, bladder, lungs, and bronchial weaknesses. Marshmallow calms nerves and increases milk flow in nursing mothers.

MILK THISTLE: Cleanses and restores the liver. Useful in hepatitis and jaundice symptoms.

MILKWEED: Helps eliminate gallstones and relieve gallbladder complaints. Aids in lung, bone, kidney and female disorders.

MINT: Soothes the intestines and removes gas.

MULLEIN: Strengthens the lungs and bronchi. Effective against pneumonia, bronchitis, hay fever, and weakened lungs. Gives pain relief, aids sleep, and removes warts.

MYRRH: Very useful in bronchial and lung disease. This was a wonderful gift from the wise men to the mother of the Christ child. Little children are prone to croup, coughs, and colds. This must have been a very highly prized herb in the days before modern medicine.

It is effective in cleansing the stomach and intestines. Myrrh has been beneficial in the fight against yeast infection and counteracting the effects of allergies and pollution. It is very effective on skin sores, sinus congestion, and infections of the mouth and throat. Removes medicines stored in body tissue.

This is another herb I would like to see in every cupboard in every household. Very safe for small children and pregnant women.

Myrrh dries mucous membrane. Certain diseases dealing with a dryness of the mucous lining would not benefit from myrrh.

NETTLE: Bladder, kidney, and urinary complaints. Helps bones, skin, lung, and thyroid disorders. Overall tonic.

OAT STRAW: Bladder, kidney, and urinary cleanser and strengthener. Helps bones.

OLIVE LEAF: Antibacterial, antifungal, antiviral. Effective against sexually transmitted disease.

OREGANO: Fresh oregano leaves chewed relieve a sore throat. Also good to relieve a nervous headache and toothache.

PARSLEY: Strengthens the endocrine system, urinary tract, liver, and spleen. Dries up milk in nursing mothers. Very high in vitamins and minerals. Helps the stomach, reduces tumors, strengthens bones, and used in weight maintenance.

PASSION FLOWER: Good for insomnia, nervous tension, and hot flashes. Decreases high blood pressure.

PAU D' ARCO: Reported to cleanse the blood and remove cancer from the system. Very good blood cleanser. Works against yeast, STD's, blood disease, liver disease, and is antibacterial.

POKE ROOT: Used as an antibiotic. Cleanses the blood and works on lymphatic, sinus, and skin infections. Effective against STDs. Clears kidney and liver congestion.

PSYLLIUM: Cleanses the bowels. Natural laxative.

PUMPKIN SEEDS: Rids intestines of parasites.

RED CLOVER: Effective blood purifier. Works against bacteria, STDs, skin, lung, and intestinal disorders. Used with weight maintenance. Strengthens bones. Reported effective against cancer.

REDMOND CLAY: There are different colors of clay: white, green, and red. Test for individual need. Pulls toxins from the body. Helps the body balance as it assists in utilizing minerals. Good poultice for skin problems.

RED RASPBERRY: Strengthens and tones the uterus. Used during pregnancy to prepare for delivery. Good for stomach problems that need an antacid. Contributes to healthy bones, hair, skin, and nails.

RHUBARB ROOT: Intestinal healing. Assists liver, gallbladder, and spleen. Relieves headaches.

ROSE HIPS: Rich in vitamin C. Fights infection and stress.

ROSEMARY: Helps relieve headaches caused by stress. Relieves symptoms of a cold, high blood pressure, and female complaints. Used in shampoo to prevent baldness.

RUE: Strengthens vision. Assists in female hormone balance. Intestinal toner.

SAFFLOWER/SAFFRON: Soothes and coats the intestinal wall. Mild diuretic and laxative. Lowers cholesterol. Removes mucous from the system. Prevents kidney stones and gout by neutralizing lactic and uric acid in the body.

SAGE: (Garden) Calming to the nerves. Eliminates headache and intestinal gas. Used in a hair rinse to relieve baldness and help hair to grow under certain conditions.

SAGE: (Wild) Great overall tonic. Calms nerves.

SANICLE: Effective against STDS. Cleanses the system of constipation and congestion.

SARSAPARILLA: Hormone-balancing herb in both male and female. Sex stimulant. Strengthens bones and nerves. Helps in hair growth. Reduces fever and clears skin disorders. Helps stomach, liver, and kidney disorders. Protects against radiation.

SASSAFRAS: Blood purifier. Male hormone stimulant. Good for stomach cramps, skin conditions, bone weakness, obesity.

SAW PALMETTO: Strengthens glandular tissue in both male and female. Especially good for prostate problems. Is beneficial for urinary problems and diabetes. Rids body of mucous in the head, sinus, and lung area.

SCULLCAP: Effective in nervous disorders. Very calming to the nerves. Relieves symptoms of head and bone aches. Helps circulation and heart muscle.

SHEPHERD'S PURSE: Useful to stop bleeding after childbirth. Also stops bleeding in lungs and from hemorrhoids. Mild diuretic.

SLIPPERY ELM: Good for many intestinal and bowel disturbances from indigestion to hemorrhoids. Helps relieve symptoms of a virus. Gelling agent that helps with bone and connective tissue strength.

SQUAW VINE: Relieves female and uterine problems.

ST. JOHN'S WORT: Overall cleansing tonic. Great for nervous disorders and depression. Helps with uterine cramps and after pains. Works on liver and kidneys.

SUMA: Boosts the immune system. Effective against stress and anemia. Hormone-balancing, mostly for women who have gone through menopause. Inhibits certain kinds of cancer.

TARRAGON: In the Middle Ages this herb was thought to increase physical strength. Pilgrims used it in their shoes before setting out on long pilgrimages. It was also used in treating the bite of a mad dog. It was taken internally for the heart, lungs, and liver.

THYME: Removes mucous from the body and settles intestines. Helps in alcoholism, hangover, and headache. Used for head and lung congestion.

TURKEY RHUBARB: Relaxes intestinal pain. Purges and cleanses the intestines.

UVA URSI: Effective in strengthening the kidneys, heart, spleen, liver, and pancreas. Used in obesity and digestive problems. Helps female complaints and works against STDs.

VALERIAN ROOT: Helps circulation, muscle cramps and nerves. Calms hysteria, epilepsy, stomach, insomnia and migraines. Reduces fevers and is useful against acne, ulcers, and arthritis. During the Dark Ages, it was noted to be useful against bruises, coughs, and plague.

WATERCRESS: Strengthens urinary tract. Good for heart disease, indigestion, and gas.

WHITE OAK BARK: Reduces enlarged veins like hemorrhoid and varicose. Helps female complaints, bladder, kidney and gallstones, enlarged thyroid, fever, liver, and skin disorders.

WHITE WILLOW BARK: An anti-inflammatory, it is effective against colds, headache, bone aches, nervous conditions, abdominal complaints, heartburn, nosebleeds, skin disorders, gangrene, and cancer.

WILD YAM: Used intestinally for colic and spasm. Strengthens liver and female hormone balance.

WINTERGREEN: Good for diabetes, bladder complaints, and skin disease. Useful in intestinal cleansing and toning and for gonorrhea. Oil is great for rheumatic complaints.

WITCH HAZEL: Branches from the witch hazel tree are used as divining rods to detect underground water. This is where they got the name, "witching rods." An effective treatment for hemorrhoids (when used in an ointment) and relief of varicose veins (applied in a warm compress). Gives topical relief for skin sores and infections.

WOOD BETONY: Good against headache, pain, and heartburn. Calms the nerves. Clears parasites. Stimulates the heart, liver, and lungs.

WORMWOOD: Expels worms. A good liniment on bruises, sprains, and swellings.

YARROW: Effective against viral complaints as it opens body pores to allow toxins to escape. Strengthens the pancreas, kidneys, and lungs. Helpful in female complaints and childhood diseases. Clears mucous out of the system. Used as a shampoo, it is reported to restore hair to the head.

YELLOW DOCK: An effective blood purifier that cleanses and tones the whole system. Clears liver, lymphatic system, lungs, and skin disorders. Works against STDs and cancer. Expels worms, and fights against anemia in the blood.

YERBA MATE: Increases immunity, energy, brain function; calms nerves; cleanses blood; used in weight control.

YUCCA: Helps with pancreas, kidney and bladder weakness, and strengthens bones and connective tissue. Yucca can be used as a shampoo and soap.

A Word of Caution

Some herbs are harmful if taken in large doses for extended lengths of time. Become informed and use much care in working with the herbs.

DIGESTIVE AIDS

The normal stomach function is to secrete hydrochloric acid to aid in digestion. If the secretion is normal, food is digested properly and there is a proper balance in the function of the stomach.

However, there are people who do not have the normal acid secretion.

1) HYPER-acidic or too much acid secreted. If this is how your stomach is, you will complain of digestive gas, bloating and gastric backwash, or even ulcers. Your personality traits will be that of one who is "hyper", or may be called a "mover and a shaker." You make the world turn with your drive and ambition. In other words you move ahead on your own and make things happen.

    For you to take a highly acidic digestive enzyme would be like pouring fuel on a fire. Best, on the other hand, to use calming products like antacids, slippery elm, and mint.

2) HYPO-acidic or not enough digestive acids secreted. You would tend to be more of a "let life happen as it might," "take it as it comes" personality. You like to move slower and are more pensive. Your rich personality gives balance and calm to the world. You are one of the peacemakers and the thinkers.

    This may be reflected in your intestinal digestion too. You don't have enough gastric acid to digest food, which makes it difficult to absorb all the nutrients from food because it is not properly broken down. Constipation and gas are more likely.

    Some digestive aids that are very useful in cases of HYPO- acidic or low gastric acid would be things like papaya, papaya/papain, hydrochloric acid, or digestive enzymes.

Other products that restore intestinal flora and maintain better balance are intestinal aids such as acidophilus, primadophilus, or bifadophilus. These are highly recommended for someone suffering with yeast infections. Individual testing will indicate which one is best and the correct amount.

Questions to ask about herbs/enzymes

Using the Bio-Kinetic checklist available at the end of the book, or the following charts for herbs for body parts, ask the following questions:

1. Do you need the herb/enzyme?

2. What herb is needed?

3. What strength or size capsule is needed?

4. How many of the herb/ enzyme are needed each day?

5. What time of day is best to take it?

6. How many days can this be taken?

Testing for herbs/enzymes:

- "Along with the vitamins and minerals you tested for, do you need herbs?" (Yes) (See following chapter on testing herbs for body parts.)

- "Do you need a digestive enzyme?" (Yes)

- "What would be the best for you? Papaya?" (No)

- "Papain?" (No)

- "Digestive enzymes?" (Yes)

- "How many do you need? One?" (No)

- "Two?" (No)

- "Three?" (Yes)

- "Do you need one with each meal?" (Yes)

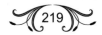

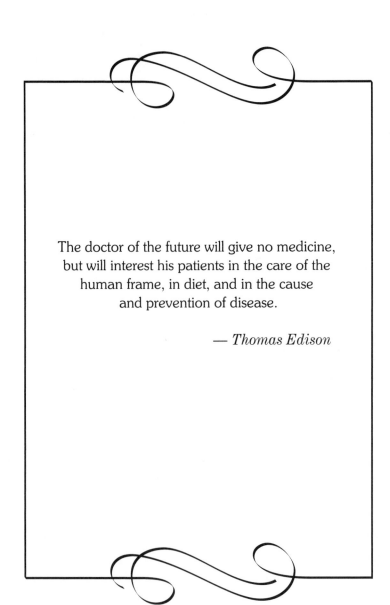

The doctor of the future will give no medicine,
but will interest his patients in the care of the
human frame, in diet, and in the cause
and prevention of disease.

— *Thomas Edison*

CHAPTER 16

Herbs Part II

POSSIBLE HERBS FOR TYPE OF INFECTION

Possible Herbs for Type of Infection Table		
VIRUS	**BACTERIA**	**YEAST**
Astragalus	Astragalus	Acidophilus
Blue Vervain	Cayenne	Bifidophilus
Burdock	Chlorophyll	Capryllic Acid
Catnip	Colloidal Silver	Cats Claw
Cats Claw	Echinacea	Chaparral
Cayenne	Garlic	Clay (White, Red, Gray)
Cleavers	Goldenseal	Colloidal Silver/Gold
Echinacea	Collodial Minerals	Colloidal Minerals
Elderberry	Myrrh	Comfrey
Feverfew	Olive Leaf	Garlic
Ginseng	Pau d' Arco	Grape Seed Extracts
Goldenseal	Peroxide	Juniper Berries
Homeopathic	Poke Root	Myrrh
Horehound	Red Clover	Olive Leaf
Hyssop	Rose hips	Pau D' Arco
Licorice Root	Other	Peroxide
Lobelia		Primadophilus
Myrrh		Tea Tree Oil
Olive Leaf		Other
Pau d' Arco		
Poke Root		
Red Clover		
Rose Hips		
Rosemary		
Sanicle		
Slippery Elm		
Uva Ursi		
White Willow		
White Oak		
Yarrow		
Yellow Dock		
Other		

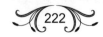

ALLERGY	STDs	PARASITE
Astragalus	Burdock	Black Walnut
Bee Propolis	Cats Claw	Borage
Bee Pollen	Chaparral	Buckthorn
Echinacea	Cleavers	Cayenne
Homeopathic Products	Comfrey	Cloves
Myrrh	Elderberry	Garlic
Rose Hips	Gotu Kola	Horsetail
Vitamin C	Hops	Horehound
Other	Olive Leaf	Male Fern
	Poke Root	Pumpkin Seeds
	Red Clover	Wood Betony
	Sanicle	Wormwood
	Uva Ursi	Yellow Dock
	Wintergreen	Other
	Yellow Dock	
	Black Walnut	
	Other	

Testing herbs for virus, yeast, bacteria, allergy and parasite:

I will do a walk through on the bacteria. All the others follow the same format:

- "Do you need astragalus for the bacteria you have?" (No)

- "Do you need echinacea for the bacteria?" (Yes)

- "How many echinacea do you need today? One?" (No)

- "Two?" (No)

- "Three?" (No

- "Four?" (Yes)

- "Five?" (No)

- "Do you want them all at once?" (No)

- "Should you take them spread out?" (Yes)

- "Do you need cayenne for the bacteria you have?" (Yes)

- "How many do you need?" "One?" (No)

- "Two?" (No)

- "Three?" (Yes)

- "Along with echinacea and cayenne, do you need garlic?" (Yes)

- "Do you want raw garlic?" (No)

- "Do you want odorless garlic?" (Yes)

- "How man capsules do you need? One?" (No)

- "Two?" (No)

- "Three?" (Yes)

- "Do you need another herb besides echinacea, cayenne, and garlic for the bacteria you have?" (Yes)

Continue testing until all the herbs needed are tested for.

If you get a "No" on the last question, you do not need to continue testing the rest of the herbs listed for bacteria.

Do this for each herb and each ailment, making note of "Yes" responses and how many are needed. I have found that it usually takes three to four herbs to treat each infection or ailment. It is possible for someone to have a virus, STDs, yeast, parasites, and allergies at the same time. (I have tested this to be the case many times.) Testing three to four herbs per infection could conceivably render you taking 20 different herbs. However, since herbs can work on more than one ailment, or overlap in their healing functions, it reduces the need for so many herbs.

Possible Herbs for Parts of the Body Table

BONES	LYMPHATIC SYSTEM IMMUNE SYSTEM SPLEEN	BRAIN/NERVES
Alfalfa	Astragalus	Black Cohosh (N)
Buckthorn	Blue Vervain	Blue Cohosh (N)
Burdock	Burdock	Blue Vervain (N)
Butchers Broom	Catnip	Borage (N)
Cats Claw	Cats Claw	Chamomile (N)
Cayenne	Cayenne	Dong Quai (N & B)
Celery Seed	Chaparral	Feverfew
Chaparral	Cleavers	Ginkgo Biloba(N & B)
Comfrey	Comfrey	Ginseng (N & B)
Dandelion	Dandelion	Goldenseal (N)
Evening Primrose	Echinacea	Gotu Kola(N & B)
Fennel	Fennel	Guarana (B)
Flaxseed	Garlic	Hawthorn (N)
Gentian	Gentian	Hops (N)
Gotu Kola	Ginseng	Kava Kava (N)
Hawthorn	Goldenseal	Kelp (N & B)
Horsetail/Shavegrass	Hyssop	Lady Slipper (N)
Hydrangea	Iceland Moss	Licorice Root (N)
Milkweed	Lobelia	Lobelia (N)
Nettle	Myrrh	Marjoram (N)
Oat Straw	Nettle	Marshmallow (N)
Poke Root	Olive Leaf	Mullein (N)
Parsley	Parsley	Oregano (N)
Red Clover	Pau d' Arco	Passion Flower (N)
Red Raspberry	Poke Root	Peppermint (N)
Safflower	Red Clover	Rosemary (N)
Sarsaparilla	Redmond Clay	Sage (N)
Sassafras	Rhubarb Root	Sarsaparilla (N)
Slippery Elm	Safflower	Scullcap (N)
Valerian Root	Sage (wild)	St. Johns Wort (N)
White Willow	Sanicle	Suma (N)
Wintergreen Oil	Sassafras	Thyme (N)
Yucca	St. John's Wort	Valerian Root (N)
	Suma	White Willow (N)
	Uva Ursi	Wood Betony (N & B)
	Valerian Root	Yerba Mate (N)
	White Willow	
	Yarrow	
	Yellow Dock	
	Yerba Mate	

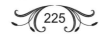

KIDNEY/BLADDER	EYES	LUNGS/BRONCHIAL
Astragalus	Eyebright	Astragalus
Buchu Leaves	Fenugreek	Barberry
Burdock	Horsetail	Blue Vervain
Butchers Broom	Rue	Borage
Cayenne		Cayenne
Chaparral		Chaparral
Cleavers	**LIVER/GALL**	Chickweed
Comfrey	**BLADDER**	Comfrey
Corn Silk	Alfalfa	Dandelion
Cranberry	Burdock	Eucalyptus
Dandelion	Cascara Sagrada	Fennel
Echinacea	Cats Claw	Fenugreek
Fennel	Celery Seed	Garlic
Ginger	Centaury	Ginger
Ginkgo Biloba	Chaparral	Ginkgo Biloba
Goldenseal	Cleavers	Ginseng
Gotu Kola	Dandelion	Goldenseal
Gravel Root	Garlic	Horehound
Horsetail	Gentian	Hyssop
Huckleberry	Gotu Kola	Licorice Root
Hydrangea	Goldenseal	Lobelia
Juniper Berries	Gravel Root	Marshmallow
Marshmallow	Hops	Milkweed
Milkweed	Milk Thistle	Mullein
Nettle	Milk Weed (GB)	Myrrh
Oat Straw	Oregon Grape Rt	Nettle
Parsley	Parsley	Red Clover
Poke Root	Pau d' Arco	Saw Palmetto
Safflower	Poke Root	Shepherd's Purse
Sarsaparilla	Rhubarb Root	Tarragon
Saw Palmetto	Sarsaparilla	Thyme
St. Johns Wort	St. John's Wort	Valerian Root
Uva Ursi	Tarragon	Wood Betony
Watercress	Uva Ursi	Yarrow
White Oak	White Oak Bark	Yellow Dock
Wintergreen	Wild Yam	
Yarrow	Wood Betony	
Yucca	Yellow Dock	
	Yerba Mate	

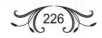
MALE ORGANS	EARS/NOSE/THROAT	HEART/ CIRCULATION
Flax seed	Astragalus	Alfalfa
Ginseng	Bayberry	Barberry
Gotu Kola	Black Walnut	Black Cohosh
Kelp	Blue Vervain	Blessed Thistle
Licorice Root	Cayenne	Blue Cohosh
Sarsaparilla	Echinacea	Butchers Broom
Sassafras	Eucalyptus	Cayenne
Saw Palmetto	Fenugreek	Celery Seed
	Garlic	Chickweed
FEMALE ORGANS	Ginseng	Comfrey
	Ginger	Dandelion
Angelica Root	Goldenseal	Dong Quai
Bayberry	Horehound	Garlic
Black Cohosh	Horsetail	Ginkgo Biloba
Blessed Thistle	Hyssop	Ginseng
Blue Cohosh	Licorice Root	Goldenseal
Blue Vervain	Lobelia	Gotu Kola
Centaurea	Myrrh	Hawthorn
Chamomile	Oregano	Licorice Root
Damiana	Pau d' Arco	Lobelia
Dong Quai	Poke Root	Passion Flower
Evening Primrose	Saw Palmetto	Pau d'Arco
False Unicorn	Slippery Elm	Rosemary
Flaxseed	Thyme	Safflower
Ginger	White Willow	Scullcap
Ginseng	Yarrow	Shepherds Purse
Gotu Kola	Yellow Dock	Suma
Horehound		Tarragon
Kelp		Uva Ursi
Licorice Root		Valerian Root
Marshmallow		Watercress
Milkweed		White Oak Bark
Parsley		Witch Hazel
Passion Flower		Wood Betony
Red Raspberry		Yellow Dock
Rosemary		
Rue		
Sarsaparilla		
Saw Palmetto		
Shepherd's Purse		
Squaw Vine		
St. John's Wort		
Suma		
Uva Ursi		
White Oak		
Wild Yam		

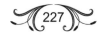

HAIR/SKIN/NAILS	STOMACH/INTESTINE	PANCREAS
Alfalfa	Alfalfa	Buchu Leaves
Bayberry	Barberry	Cedar Berries
Blue Vervain	Black Walnut	Chromium
Borage	Buckthorn	Comfrey
Buckthorn	Cascara Sagrada	Ginseng
Burdock	Catnip	Huckleberry
Cayenne	Cats Claw	Juniper Berries
Chaparral	Cayenne	Licorice Root
Chickweed	Chamomile	Saw Palmetto
Cleavers	Chickweed	Uva Ursi
Comfrey	Cloves	Wintergreen
Dandelion	Comfrey	Yarrow
Echinacea	Fennel	Yucca
Evening Primrose	Fenugreek	
Flaxseed	Garlic	**ENDOCRINE SYSTEM**
Garlic	Gentian	Alfalfa
Goldenseal	Ginger	Bladderwrack
Horsetail/Shavegrass	Ginseng	Buchu Leaves
Jojoba	Goldenseal	Cayenne
Kelp	Hops	Chamomile
Mullein	Horsetail	Chickweed
Myrrh	Licorice Root	Dandelion
Nettle	Mint	Dulse
Oat Straw	Myrrh	Ginseng
Plantain	Parsley	Gotu Kola
Poke Root	Psyllium Husks	Guarana
Red Clover	Pumpkin Seeds	Huckleberry
Redmond Clay	Red Clover	Iceland Moss
Red Raspberry	Red Raspberry	Irish Moss
Rosemary	Rue	Kelp
Sage	Safflower	Licorice Root
Sarsaparilla	Sanicle	Nettle
Sassafras	Slippery Elm	Parsley
Slippery Elm	Sarsaparilla	Poke Root
Valerian Root	Sassafras	Red Clover
White Oak Bark	Thyme	Redmond Clay
White Willow	Turkey Rhubarb	Sassafras
Wintergreen	Uva Ursi	Saw Palmetto
Witch Hazel	Valerian Root	Uva Ursi
Wormwood	Watercress	White Oak
Yarrow	White Willow	
Yellow Dock	Wild Yam	
Yucca	Wintergreen	
	Wood Betony	
	Wormwood	

Herbal Formulas Index

CHAPTER 17

Herbal Formulas

As a general rule, I don't recommend ready-made herbal formulas. One or two herbs in the formula that are not compatible with your body, will negate the whole formula.

One person can take an herbal formula and do just great with it. Someone else will take it and be "wired" or "depressed" or it does "nothing" for them. Individual make-up is the reason we would be well to customize our own formulas.

Test to see if a ready-made formula is good for you.

Steps to making herbal formulas:

1) Test for the herbs needed in the formula you intend to make. Write the name of each one down on a piece of paper.

2) Purchase the herbs in a powdered form. Most health food stores carry herbs in bulk or powdered form. If you do not have a health food store that does so, then herbs can be ordered by mail with a small fee for shipping and handling. I have used San Francisco Herb company and have been pleased with their products and services.

San Francisco Herb and Natural Food Company
47444 Kato Road
Fremont, California 94538

3) Test for tablespoon amounts of each herb. Read the name of each herb and ask, "How many tablespoons of _____ do I need in this formula?" Count and test for amounts and write it by each herb tested. This is your "recipe."

4) Measure the herbs into a bowl or jar and mix together.

5) From this mix, you will then test for the number of capsules or teaspoons needed each day.

The following formulas are suggestions ONLY. No claim is made that they are the exact ones for you. Always ask to see if another herb might be needed that is not on the list.

Herbal capsules are safe to store on a shelf away from heat or direct sunlight.

Store liquid herbs or formulas in a refrigerator to help keep the product stable.

**Remember that for anything of a serious nature, consult a health-care professional.

ACNE

Test for HAIR/SKIN/NAILS herbs under HERBS FOR BODY PARTS.

Test to see if the acne is caused from hormone changes, bacteria or yeast in the skin, improper skin care, or stress.

If the cause is hormone changes, adjust the hormone herbs for male or female. If the acne is because of a problem with yeast or bacteria in the skin, test for skin care products available on the market. If it is from improper skin care or touching the skin with the hands, teach skin care techniques. If acne is stress-related, herbs for hormones and nerves will help. Other things that help the skin are zinc, potassium, vitamin C.

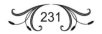

APPENDICITIS

Symptoms include a sharp pain in lower right abdominal area. Appendicitis indicates an inflammation of the appendix whether viral, bacterial, yeast, or food irritation.

If fever or vomiting occur, see a doctor immediately.

ARTHRITIS, RHEUMATISM, GOUT

Test for herbs for BONES and NERVES under HERBS FOR BODY PARTS. Test for amounts of each herb and how many capsules.

BLOOD PURIFIER/BODY CLEANSING FORMULA

Milk Thistle	Burdock	Yellow Dock	Cats Claw
Echinacea	Sarsaparilla	Goldenseal	Borage
Psyllium Husks	Garlic	Chaparral	Yerba Mate
Dandelion	Ginseng	Poke Root	
Ginger	Cleavers	Licorice	
Slippery Elm	Red Clover	Kelp	

Test for which herbs are most beneficial for your body. Mix powdered herb in a jar. Test for number of capsules to be taken each day.

BRUISING LINIMENT

Muscle sprains, bruises, connective tissue injury.

Equal parts each: prickly ash, goldenseal, calendula flower, ginseng, myrrh gum, hyssop, cinnamon, cayenne

Soak 3½ oz. powdered herb mix in 1 quart apple cider vinegar. Let this set in a warm dark place (closet) for two weeks. Shake every day.

To use this, apply with a gauze or cloth saturated with formula.

Store in a cool, dark pantry. Best if used within a year.

COLDS, FLU, FEVERS

Test for mixture of virus herbs (Chapter 15); mix and test for number of capsules needed. Follow with a warm bath. Add 2 TBS ginger or ½ cup apple cider vinegar to the bath water.

COUGH FORMULA

One spring, due to the high occurrence of coughs and an increase in the Respiratory Virus, I decided to concentrate on a formula to help my family should they come down with the cough. I had these herbs growing in my yard, so I tested for amounts of each green herb and made this wonderful cough formula. I have shared it with others who have found it to be an effective formula.

4 large comfrey leaves   40 fresh garlic greens
7 large mullein leaves   8—10 parsley branches
4 large echinacea leaves   8—10 fennel branches
10 horehound leaves

Stuff the herbs in a jar. Cover with apple cider vinegar. Shake every day, two or three times, for 2 weeks. (Keep it on the window sill while it is processing.) Strain. Add honey and glycerin to taste. Refrigerate and use within a year.

EPSTEIN-BARR FORMULA

1 liter White Wine

Bring to boil. Boil 3–5 minutes.

Remove from heat. Add Wormwood as tested for. Guideline is 3 TBS. chopped herb or 1 TBS. powdered herb.

Let cool. Strain if desired. Store in refrigerator.

Test for amount to be used. Guideline: 4 tablespoons per day for adults; less for children. Test for how many days. This works fast on the virus.

ESSIAC FORMULA

Blood cleansing formula

Burdock 10 ½ oz.
 Turkey Rhubarb ½ oz.
Sheep Sorrell 8 oz.
Slippery Elm 2 oz.

Mix powdered herbs in container. Test for number of capsules to be taken each day.

EYEWASH

Tired eyes. Eye strain.

1 part each: goldenseal, eyebright, bayberry, raspberry leaf

Mix. Make a tea with 1 teaspoon herb in one-half pint of boiling water. Cool. Refrigerate. Discard after 1 week.

HEMORRHOID

Witch Hazel liquid applied directly with gauze pad.

OR

Equal parts Witch Hazel leaves, Bayberry Bark, Goldenseal. Mix and add to Olive Oil to form a paste. Apply directly.

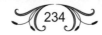

OR

Test for number (Usually 4—6) Cayenne Pepper capsules/day.

OR

1 part Dandelion	1 part Cascara Sagrada
1 part Chicory	1 part Oregon Grape Root
½ part Licorice	1 part Cayenne Pepper

Test for right amounts for your body and number of capsules to take internally.

HERPES FORMULA

Echinacea	Oregon Grape Root	Yellow Dock	Lysine
Chaparral	Licorice	Burdock	
Sarsaparilla	Ginger	Dandelion	
Gravel Root	Sanicle	Hops	

Test for tablespoon amount of which herbs would be best for your body. Mix them all together then test for capsules needed each day.

INSOMNIA

Insomnia can be caused by many things. Test to see if the underlying reason is emotional trauma; infection in the nervous system; physical trauma to the head or nerves; physical ailments that cause pain or difficulty breathing; hidden angers or fears; recent death or loss; a body full of caffeine or stimulants of any kind.

With emotional fears, traumas, angers or losses, it is best to see a counselor to uncover the hidden causes.

If the problem is physical, test the herbs for the body part that is affected. This might include herbs for nerves, bones, lungs, and brain.

KIDNEY and GALLSTONES

Dandelion	Marshmallow
Gravel Root	Ginger
Parsley	Licorice
Lemon Balm	Bayberry
Lobelia	Cayenne

Test for tablespoon amount of each herb, number of capsules, or liquid drops of each herb in distilled water.

Test to see if your body would do better with herbal capsules or liquid herbs. Liquid herbs are more readily available by the body and enter the blood stream faster. Bulk herbs are subject to the action of the digestive enzymes and work through the digestive system.

Other suggestions:
- Tumeric is good for removing kidney and gallstones.

- Drink nothing but water off boiled onions.

- Drink a six pack of Coke and follow it with a can of asparagus.

Drink distilled water and alternate with lemon juice. At the end of the day, take a tablespoon of olive oil. This greases the tubes so the stones can slip through easily.

LIVER AILMENTS AND INDIGESTION

Gentian	Golden Seal	Cats Claw
Oregon Grape Root	Dandelion	Borage
Cascara Sagrada	Wild Yam	Gravel Root
Lobelia	Ginger	Yerba Mate
Licorice	Milk Thistle	

Fill "OO" size capsules. Take 2—3 times/day with warm water just before each meal. Test which of these herbs are best, or test from the LIVER or STOMACH list under HERBS FOR BODY PARTS.

MENSTRUAL CRAMPS

Consider testing for:

Kava Kava, White Willow

1 part Ginger	2 parts Cramp Bark
1 part Lobelia	1 part Chamomile
2 parts Angelica/or Dong Quai	2 Parts Raspberry leaves
2 parts Squawvine	2 parts Peppermint

Mix 6 ounces of powdered herb mix in 1 quart apple cider vinegar. Let this stand for 1 day. Shake it occasionally. Strain. Refrigerate. Use 1 TBS. 3 times/day as needed for cramps.

MORNING SICKNESS

Accept the pregnancy. Rejection of baby increases sickness.

Catnip/Fennel tea. Take 15 drops every hour with nausea

Keep bowels clean with high-fiber foods. Do not use strong bowel herbs, or colonics.

Ginger tea or chewing ginger pieces help.

OINTMENTS, WASHES, POULTICES, HERBAL FIRST AID

This is very concentrated. Use herbal oil blends for this. One to two drops at a time is usually sufficient to relieve colds, flu, headache, pain, sprains, depression.

Blend: cinnamon, olive oil, thyme, eucalyptus, camphor, marjoram, lemon balm

Mix the oils into a blend and store in an airtight container. Rub on the skin over pressure points you test for.

Store in a pantry.

PASTE

Used for burns, fractures, sprains and cuts, infection, swelling

3 parts comfrey leaves or root   1 part lobelia
½ part wheat germ oil   ½ part honey
1 part cayenne   1 part marshmallow

Mix all together. Store in a jar with wide mouth for easy access. Apply to skin freely. Cover with gauze.

Store in cool, dark pantry.

PLAGUE FORMULA

Just for fun I have to include this story and formula.

The story is told about the plague formula that dates back to the Middle Ages and the days of the black plague.

There was a group of individuals who came up with this formula and took it faithfully. They never contracted the plague, but availed themselves the opportunity of going into the homes of those who suffered with the disease and were too weak to get out of bed. Under these circumstances, the formula users were able to relieve the dead and dying of their jewels and precious belongings.

The thing that makes it appealing to me is the fact that there are many plagues that inflict man, and if this worked for the black plague, there is some merit in knowing how to make formulas for modern day plagues. Perhaps some of these very herbs will be invaluable in our modern day fight against the diseases we face in the form of yeast, bacteria, Epstein Barr Virus, chickenpox, measles, etc.

This is not claimed to be a cure-all. Test and see if it would benefit you or your family.

This is best used as a liquid formula. Mix the following liquid ingredients:

8 parts apple cider vinegar
5 parts honey
2 parts comfrey root
1 part lobelia leaf/seed
1 part marshmallow root
1 part oak bark
1 part uva ursi, hydrangea, or gravel root

5 parts glycerine U.S.P.
2 parts garlic juice, fresh
1 part wormwood
1 part black walnut bark
1 part mullein leaf
1 part scullcap

To make concentrates

Each herb should be made into a concentrate individually. Start by soaking the herb for four hours or more in enough distilled water to cover it completely. After soaking, add more distilled water so that the total equals 16 oz. (.5 liter) water per 4 oz. (113 grams) herb. Use a multiple of these amounts for a larger quantity of formula. Using these amounts, approximately one gallon (3.75 liters) of formula will be produced.

After adding the appropriate amount of distilled water to the soaked herb (use distilled water for the purpose of purity), simmer the herb on very low heat in a covered pan or double boiler for 30 minutes. Strain the liquid into a clean pan. Put the liquid into a double boiler or on very low heat (uncovered) and simmer (steam) it down to one-fourth of the original volume (4 oz. 125 ml.) Only after all ingredients have been prepared should the liquids be mixed.

DO NOT USE ALUMINUM, TEFLON, OR CRACKED PORCELAIN. Glass, corning ware, or stainless steel are best.

Dose: 1 tsp. 3 times a day; or 1 tablespoon every half hour if infected.

Refrigerate and discard after a year.

SUNBURN TREATMENT

One summer I had a friend who spent too long on the beach in the sun. Being fair skinned, she burned badly.

When I saw her condition, I came home and tested for herbs that could be mixed to relieve her pain and the burn she was feeling.

This is the mix we came up with. She dipped a gauze strip in the formula and kept applying it until the sunburn had healed.

The formula has since been used by family members when needed.

1 cup apple cider vinegar	½ cup Aloe Vera Juice
3—5 medium comfrey leaves	800 IU capsule vitamin E

Blend in blender. Apply with gauze and leave on burn. Reapply as necessary.

Discard any unused portion.

WEIGHT-MAINTENANCE PROGRAM

Iceland/Irish Moss	Nettle	Cayenne
Bladderwrack	Wild Yam	Chickweed
Wild Cherry Bark	Peppermint	Rhubarb Root
Sarsaparilla	Dandelion	Saffron
Fennel	Kava Kava	Rue
Cedar Berries	Kola Nut	Guarana
Red Clover	Parsley	Uva Ursi
Sassafras	Licorice Root	Yellow Dock

1) Test which of these herbs are best for your body.

2) Test to see if there are other herbs you need to mix with these.

3) Test for the tablespoon amount of each herb.

4) Just like you would follow a recipe, mix the herbs together in a bowl or jar.

5) Test for the number of capsules you need to take each day from the mix.

Since these herbs do give energy, it is best not to take them at bedtime.

The herbs in this formula will be effective for a few weeks and will need to be re-tested and adjusted regularly.

When I did my formula, it needed to be changed after three weeks. The herbs had been very effective in strengthening my endocrine system. I now test for other herbs that will facilitate healing in other organs.

This program is not a get slim quick scheme. This will be like running a marathon as opposed to a 100 yard dash. You are very familiar with the yo-yo weight programs in which you lose fast, you gain it back fast. The intent of this weight maintenance is to form solid habits and strengthen the inner core before seeing much result in weight reduction.

As the endocrine system heals, the metabolism increases, energy levels improve and then the body is able to burn off excess fat.

Too many diet plans rob the process because they give a pseudo-replacement for inner body strength. Weight maintenance must be based on firm principles and not short cuts.

This is a four-step program:

1)   Take the formula and re-adjust as needed

2)   Exercise. Test for how many minutes/day you need.

3)   Diet. Cut back either fat, sugar, or portion size.

4)   Reason. Everyone needs a good reason. It needs to be something very meaningful either for yourself or someone else. Some ideas might be looking good in a bikini next summer, look good for the class reunion, impress husband or boyfriend, prove something to someone (even self) that you are capable to such a change.

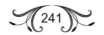

YEAST-CLEANSING FORMULA

8 oz. Water   1 TBS. Liquid clay/or 1 tsp. Powder clay
                            (Test for white, gray, or green)

Mix together then break 1 capsule capryllic acid into the mix.

2 capsules acidophilus. Break 1 into the mix, swallow the other.

1 heaping tsp. Psyllium husks

Mix in a blender. Drink quickly.

Follow with 8 oz water. Take at bedtime.

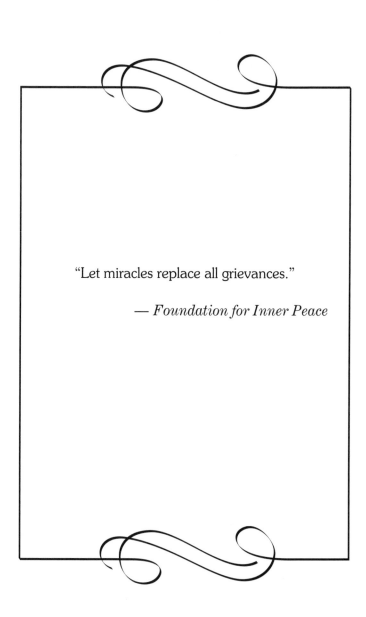

"Let miracles replace all grievances."

— *Foundation for Inner Peace*

CHAPTER 18

Frequently Asked Questions

Did I come down with a cold when I was on these herbs?

No. Herbs trigger a cleanse. Cleansing symptoms include all of those of a head cold, a flu, stomach flu, a bad hangover, intense pain, or griping anywhere in any body part. It's good to feel this, for it means the herbs are working.

One of my clients got very sick a few days after starting the herbal cleanse. Her husband rushed her to the hospital where hundreds of dollars worth of tests were run. They found nothing medically wrong with her. She woke up the next morning feeling just great. She called and said, "That must have been the cleanse you were telling me about."

Most people experience a cleanse of some kind. You may feel extreme symptoms, or you may cleanse mildly. No one method of cleansing is right or wrong. It will be just right for your system.

How do you feel about enemas?

Enemas are a great healing tool IF the person tests for and needs them. Enemas must be done with care to not puncture the colon. Especially use caution with children.

When we play outside and get dirt on our hands, we come in and wash it off. When we get "dirt" inside, we do an enema to wash it out. This "dirt"

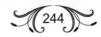

could be virus, yeast, bacteria, parasites, undesirable foods that need to be flushed, or an impacted or collapsed colon.

Instructions:

Most pharmacies have hot-water bottle kits. This is a hot water bottle with a tube and two or three different tips.

The flared tip is for douching; the straight tip is for enemas.

Disposable enemas are available but the preferred way to cleanse a colon is with tap water.

Fill the bag with tepid water (tepid means comfortable when run on the wrist over the pulse site). This is how a mother tests the temperature of her baby's bottle. If it is the right temperature on the wrist, it will be the right temperature inside the body.

Lubricate the end of the tip, then insert it into the rectum and un-clamp the tube.

Allow the water to run until you feel the urge to expel it. Close the clamp and go to the toilet!!

Repeat this until two or three bags of water have been used. The healthy adult colon should hold one full bag of water.

The best position is to kneel on the floor with the chest resting on the floor in front of you. This allows the water to run into the folds of the large intestine. Gravity will allow for better water flow.

Herbs can be added to the water if you test for them. The most common herbs are garlic, myrrh, and ginger.

What is the ileocecal valve?

This valve is located at the joining site between the small and large intestine. It's purpose is to close after food has passed from the small to large bowel, which keeps the material from "back washing" into the small intestine.

If this valve gets stuck open, it causes gas, nausea, pain in the lower right abdominal area, (similar to appendicitis), ringing in ears, and dizziness.

It helps to reflex the colon. Here is one method that is very effective.

1) Starting just under the rib cage on the left hand side, take the tips of the fingers and press in gently. Hold it for a few seconds.

2) Next, move to your waist line on the left, just between the hip and rib cage. Press in and hold the site for a few seconds.

3) Press inside the prominent hip bone on the left, going in at an angle to get your fingers just inside the hip bone. Hold firmly for a few seconds and then release.

4) Moving to the right side of the body, do a mirror reflection of the left side only in reverse. Press your finger tips inside the right hip joint, hold and release.

5) Waist level on the right side is the next site. Press down with your fingertips, hold and release.

6) Just under the rib cage on the right side completes the circle.

Repeat this pattern as many times as you test for.

To adjust the ileocecal valve, place your fingertips to the right, just below the naval. Press in deep and firm with

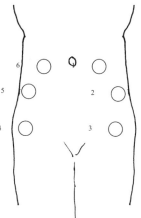

Pressure points to reflex the colon

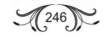

downward pressure towards the right leg. By doing this, you allow the valve to be held open and release any debris that may be keeping it from closing.

After holding that site for a few seconds, move the fingertips to the right hip joint area just over the appendix. Push in firmly but gently pulling the muscle of the abdomen in an upwards stroke towards the left shoulder. This picks up the large intestine and allows the valve to close.

Hold this position for a few seconds, then release slowly.

This can be repeated as often as necessary to train the valve to remain shut.

What causes headaches?

One of the main causes of headaches is stress. We each have a particular organ that responds to stress, and stress is expressed physically according to the function of that organ.

Organ That Manifests Your Stress	
ORGAN	SYMPTOMS OF STRESS
Brain	Forgetfulness, headaches, fuzziness or confusion in the head, inability to concentrate, possibly lead to strokes or brain weakness later in life.
Heart	Pain in the chest, heaviness or pressure over the heart, Skipping of beats, palpitations, shortness of breath, which can lead to possible heart problems in the future.
Stomach	Heart burn, indigestion, stomach pain, gas, nausea, over secretion of gastric acids which creates the need for constant ingestion of antacids. Can eventually lead to ulcers
Nervous system	Headaches, irritability, depression, anxiety, numbness in the face, hands or feet, neck and shoulder tension, feels like tight bands around the head, dizziness, nausea, overuse of antidepressants, fibromyalgia
Large Intestine	Colitis, spastic colon, gas, pain, cramping in lower bowel, nausea, indigestion.
Adrenal glands	Hyperactivity, nervousness, always on the go, can't relax, low back ache over the kidney/adrenal area. Can cause the body to wear out faster.

Other causes of headache can include such things as bones in the neck being out of alignment, Epstein-Barr, yeast, bacteria, or allergies in the nervous system or brain, overuse of stimulants, trauma or stress to the nerves. Test for the cause of the headache, then take appropriate action to rid the system of infections with proper supplementation if the cause deals with infections. If the headaches result from stress or trauma, accupuncture, hypnotherapy, or meditation would be recommended. One of the more common causes is the neck bones out of alignment.

One of my clients told me that he had migraines from as early as he could remember. His parents spent a lot of time and money trying to find the cause, but to no avail. After he got married, his wife recommended he go see a chiropractor.

The two bones at the top of his spine were out of alignment, which pinched nerves going to his head. Once those were popped into place his headaches ceased. Sometime later he was carrying a set of two by fours up some stairs by balancing them on his head. He felt his neck pop out of alignment and a new headache begin.

Due to his previous experience, it was easy to acknowledge the source of his headaches.

How long until I feel better?

The length of time it takes to heal depends on several things: the strength of your immune system, inherited genetic strengths, and on how many different illnesses there are that need to be cleansed from your system. On the average it takes four to six weeks. However, it may take longer than that to regain total health. Your body has to adjust to a new level of a health experience. It will be like forming a habit of healthy thinking.

Now that I am well, will I stay this way?

The struggle to keep your body healthy and fit seems to be one of life's challenges. Each time illness strikes, you learn something new. If you view disease as a chance to learn something, then it will have been worth it.

We could say illness is a wake-up call to the immune system. Compare this to our military forces. When we are involved in war, the military becomes alert and active, working together for a common cause.

During times of peace, they get a little lax and let their guard down. They begin to experience boredom and restlessness.

The immune system is our first line of defense. An invading virus, allergy, or bacteria will actually strengthen you if the enemy is not too overpowering.

Give the military the right tools they need during war time and they do a great job. Give the immune system the right tools it needs during an invasion, and you get the same result.

Many tools are used in a days time to accomplish various tasks. Choosing the right tool helps you do a better job. For instance, if you want to pound a nail into a wall, the handle of a screwdriver or a rolling pin work just fine, but if you want to do the job in the most efficient manner then a hammer is the tool to use.

Using Bio-Kinetic testing skills will give you the right tools to maintain health in the most efficient way.

Will I always be on herbs and vitamins?

Herbs heal. When they have done their job you use them only as you test for them to maintain health.

Compare herbs to crutches. When you break a leg, you use a crutch. When your leg is healed, you discard the crutch. When the virus, bacteria, parasite, yeast or stress is overcome, you will discontinue certain herbs.

This is where Bio-Kinetic testing is important. Where one individual needs to drop an herb, another will test to stay on a low dosage for maintenance. For example, someone who is plagued with allergies will stay on Echinacea or a similar immune- boosting herb; however, if your immune system is strong, you need to use this type of herb only occasionally.

What causes arthritis?

There are four schools of thought on arthritis:

1) The medical field describes arthritis as an inflammation of the bones and/or joints.

2) Some believe there is an inherited tendency. If arthritis runs in your family line, you are pre-programmed for it. Do all you can to exercise, watch your diet and take supplements to turn the tide in your favor.

3) Another thought is that your body lacks vital nutrients. If this is the case, test for the necessary minerals and herbs to correct it.

4) Others feel arthritis is the result of holding onto resentments, angers, hostility, rigid thought patterns, and criticism.

When Jesus Christ taught us to love our enemy and do good to those who spitefully use us, He did not say it for the benefit of the enemy. We pay a high price with our own physical health if we hang on to resentments and angers towards another. Forgiving others and ourselves is one of the best healing formulas known to relieve many of life's physical (emotional, spiritual AND mental) illnesses.

I have poor bladder control. What can I do?

Women tend more to a weakness in the bladder than men, due to the placement of the sex organs. Pregnancy, a tipped, or a swollen uterus will put pressure on the bladder, which over time will cause poor urinary control.

There are a couple of exercises that help with urinary muscle weakness. This is effective for both male and female.

When you feel the urge to urinate, take your time and walk *slowly* to the bathroom. If you have a small bladder or poor muscle control, this will begin to stretch the bladder and strengthen muscle tone.

Someone who has a small bladder could visualize his bladder as growing bigger and bigger, just like a balloon that is inflated.

Try this exercise: Release some urine into the toilet, use the muscle sphincter around the bladder to stop the flow, urinate some more, then stop the flow. Repeat this until the bladder is empty. This adds muscle tone and more bladder control.

Walking is a great exercise to strengthen the muscles around the bladder.

Possible causes of enuresis can be both physical or emotionally based. Physical causes such as Epstein-Barr virus, yeast or herpes in the bladder or prostate, chronic infections in the kidney, and parasites are known to trigger bed wetting.

Emotional causes for bladder complaints are subconsciously verbalized with: "I am pissed off at someone."

Sex abuse in early childhood also triggers the body's memory of a "wet feeling" in the crotch.

I worked with a young man who was 17 years old and still wet the bed. He wanted to go with a high school sports team to another state for competitions. He didn't feel he could because of his embarrassing secret.

During a color hypnotherapy session, we found his problems stemmed back to when he was a three-year-old child with a possessive mother. Subconsciously he was controlling her by wetting his pants and bed.

Luckily he resolved this and was able to go on and participate with his team in interstate competitions.

My baby is feverish and pulling his ears. What causes this?

Allergies, infection, and teething are causes of irritation in the ears of an infant.

Teething causes a variety of symptoms. We learn very fast on our own children. When my first baby was about eight months old, she had diarrhea, a diaper rash, a fever, and a runny nose. She was fussy, irritable and pulling at her ears. I assumed there was a bad infection so I took her to the doctor and got an antibiotic. (This was before I knew much about herbs.)

She continued with the symptoms even after the antibiotic was gone. A few days later she woke up smiling with a shining new tooth on the bottom gum. All the symptoms of "infection" went away as mysteriously as they had come on.

Watching my other children, I became aware that teething does cause them much grief.

Allergies, bacteria, and viruses also cause a child to pull at his ears. This would be considered an infection. Test to see if it is viral or bacterial. Remember that antibiotics do not work on viruses.

Why do I always get pneumonia when I am sick?

The weakest organ of your body is where infection tends to settle. For instance, if your lungs have been weakened by a previous illness such as pneumonia, hay fever, or allergies they will be an easy target for any current infection. This same principle applies to any body organ.

It is a good idea to test which organ is the weakest organ, then test for herbs from the HERBS FOR BODY PARTS list to take until the organ has been strengthened.

Why can't I test when I am not feeling well?

When your energy is down, it makes it more difficult to test someone else because it takes energy to test. If you do not feel well, say, "I don't have the energy right now. I will test you tomorrow?"

The more you test and work with energy, the more your energy level will increase. This is very much like exercising a muscle in your body. The more you work at an exercise program, the stronger your muscles become.

There have been times when I worked all day on other people, only to have one of my children come and ask to be tested. I needed time to rest

for a few minutes before I could test them. Or, I'd tell them that I was too tired, could they please wait until tomorrow. They understand when I communicate that to them.

Remember, this is a new experience for you. It is not wise to run faster than you have strength. Start slow, but practice each day. Your endurance and ability will increase as you get used to using the energy fields available to you.

I am going in for surgery. What vitamins and herbs should I take?

Things to test for pre-op are: vitamin E, calcium, multiple vitamins/minerals, cayenne pepper, echinacea, myrrh, or yarrow.

Post-Op: vitamin E, vitamin C, calcium, multiple vitamins/minerals, cayenne pepper, yarrow, garlic. (Echinacea and myrrh should be used only AFTER the antibiotic is discontinued if one is used.)

Myrrh helps clean out anesthesia or other medicines used for a short time to facilitate the surgery.

Test herbs for specific organs that were operated on from the list: "Herbs for body parts." For instance, if the bones are operated on, test for herbs that can be taken to promote more rapid healing in the bones.

There are two things I suggest someone NOT take a few days before surgery: Vitamin C and garlic. These two products thin the blood. Again, test the individual because they may need vitamin C to help strengthen against infection, but be sure to ask, "Will this thin your blood too much?"

How often should I do a parasite treatment?

Parasite cleansing herbs as tested for are used for two weeks straight. After that, they should be used every time you travel out of your local residence. You should come home and test for parasites and the herbs that will get rid of them. The recommended amount is usually four a day, two in the morning and two at night, for three or four days after any trip.

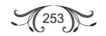

If you go on an extended trip that lasts more than two or three days, then it is a good idea to take the herbs morning and night the whole time you are gone. I have worked with couples who have gone on foreign tours and taken their parasite herbs faithfully. Upon returning from the trip, beaming with joy they call to say, "Everyone else got sick, but we had a wonderful time!!"

If you have a pet in your home, you need to repeat the parasite herbs every week for two days in a row. This applies mostly to dogs, cats, lizards, and snakes. Birds, fish, and rabbits don't seem to pass as many parasites on to humans.

Why do I use different herbs each time for the same illness?

The herbs you test for will vary according to which organ is affected by an illness.

With any good military strategy, we want to be able to surprise the enemy. If a general used the exact same war plan each time, the enemy would anticipate his maneuvers and never be defeated.

Viruses are coded genetically different from bacteria and parasites. Epstein-Barr settles in different organs each time which will manifest different symptoms.

Because a different organ is affected with each illness, and because each disease is coded different, the healing herbs will change to adapt to the situation. Remember that each organ responds to a different herb for healing.

What is a quick fix for a sprain?

My boys have been involved in athletic programs for years. It is impossible to avoid sprains and pulled muscles that come with such activities.

Several years ago while treating one of the many injuries, a nursery rhyme from years ago came into my mind:

Jack and Jill went up the hill to fetch a pail of water.
Jack fell down and broke his crown, and Jill came tumbling after.
Up Jack got, and home did trot, as fast as he could caper
To Old Dame Dob, who patched his knob with vinegar and brown paper.

This is a healing tool that has been passed down for generations in a child's rhyme. They didn't have gauze or paper towels, so they used brown paper.

Put apple cider vinegar on a folded paper towel, tissue, or gauze product, apply it directly to a pulled or sprained muscle, and leave it overnight. If it is an arm or leg that has been injured, an ace wrap can be used over the paper towel or disposable tissue to help hold it in place.

Or, put a cup of vinegar in a tub of warm water. This helps relieve sore, aching muscles in any part of the body.

What is the best water to use?

The water on this earth is not found in a pure unpolluted state. I have clients who back packed for twenty miles to an oasis to be able to drink water from a fresh source. They got intestinal parasites from the water.

Our city water is treated with chemicals to destroy infectious diseases. Chemicals are a source of health problems to many who are sensitive or allergic to them.

One of my daughters is allergic to chlorine. She has never drunk much water. When we found her allergy to be to the chlorine in the water, we started buying her bottled water. She is drinking more water and feeling healthier. Water is a invaluable in cleansing and flushing impurities from the body.

You can buy water purifiers, filters or home water treatment programs. Or, you can purchase water from companies that sell purified water.

Distilled water is the best water to use with a cleansing program for it is a hungry water that pulls toxins from the body. There are some very good reverse osmosis units available now on the market that run a close second to distilled in their removal of all contaminants from the drinking water.

What herbs can I take during pregnancy?

A growing fetus needs a chance to get established. For this reason, you should never use strong cleansing herbs in the first three months.

Herbs that test to be safe for most women are: slippery elm for virus, myrrh for head congestion, raspberry leaf for the uterus, alfalfa for vital vitamins and minerals or a pre-natal vitamin (whichever one they test for), ginger and/or B6 for morning sickness, vitamin C for healthy cell formation, calcium for bones and teeth, and nettle for allergies, iron and over all tonic.

Homeopathic products, essential oils, essences and perfumes can be used as they are tested for.

My neighbor was having a hard time going into labor. She tested to drink a quart of raspberry leaf and take capsules of blue cohosh. She had a natural delivery without having her labor induced.

Another client has 19 children. I met her after the birth of her 18th baby. She did not have an easy delivery because her uterus was stretched out after so many pregnancies.

Her 19th pregnancy was the first time she had used herbs. She saw me frequently for testing and adjusting of herbs during the nine month pregnancy. At the time of delivery, her doctor had anesthesiologists and surgeons standing by in anticipation of a caesarean section.

She declared this to be the easiest delivery with the fastest recovery she had ever experienced.

The right herbs make a big difference in the natural delivery process.

There are certain things that go different than we expect during delivery, which will change the course of the delivery. No herb on earth can prevent a breach delivery or change the shape of a woman's pelvis to be big enough to deliver if she is anatomically small.

Under normal circumstances, herbs are an asset during pregnancy.

How do I get rid of warts?

There are several things that have been used. Test for or try different ones that will work for you.

1) Use a pin or needle and work into the wart to loosen it up. Apply cayenne pepper and a band-aid. Each day clean off the scab that will form. Reapply cayenne and a band-aid until the wart pulls out with the new scab. Cayenne burns out the roots of a wart.

2) Tape a slice of garlic over the wart. Wear it overnight. Do this as many nights as needed until the wart has turned black and dried up.

3) Pound a mullein leaf into a poultice. Apply and hold in place with a cloth or ace wrap.

4) Getting the wart burned off by a medical doctor destroys the roots and gets rid of a wart quickly.

What causes dizziness?

The main causes of dizziness include the following:

1) Infections in the inner ear such as yeast, virus, or bacteria.

2) Allergies are a major contributing factor. It could be the seasonal pollens, a food you are eating, or something in the air that you breathe, such as the chemical from factory pollutants. If this is the case, then the dizziness could persist off and on all year.

3) Certain prescription medications.

4) Stenosis, decay, or hardening of the inner ear bones, or increased fluid retention in the semicircular canals such as one might see in arthritis or Meniere's disease.

Herbs for infection, homeopathic remedies, ginkgo biloba, extra calcium, magnesium, and manganese have been used successfully in most cases.

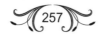

What is carpal tunnel and what can I do for it?

The nerves in the wrist pass through a small opening in the wrist bones. With repeated trauma to these nerves through the years by active use of the wrists, the nerves can become swollen and cause pain, numbness, and tingling in the wrists and hands.

Typists, piano players, gymnasts, jack-hammer employees, mechanics, and postal sorters are just a few examples of those who may be at risk to develop carpal tunnel syndrome.

One suggestion that I have found to be very effective in preventing or reducing the symptoms of this is to wear a wrist brace until the symptoms go away. The brace should be made from leather or canvas. Do not use any material that stretches or gives when the wrist is bent. Cut a strip of leather or canvas 1½ –2" wide (depending o the length of your wrist) and long enough to go around your wrist with enough overlapping to sew some velcro strips on to hold the brace in place. This is to be worn day and night (removing only to shower). If this is not effective after two to three weeks and the pain persists, go see your doctor.

Taking additional vitamin B6 (As you test for it) at bedtime helps with nerve restoration.

What Causes Ulcers?

An ulcer is described as an irritation to the lining of the stomach or intestinal walls. Ulcers have been located in the stomach, and the small and the large intestines.

The more common cause of ulcers is stress. More recent studies indicate that ulcers may be caused from bacterium. Bio-Kinetic testing will reveal the cause and help determine the approach to clear up the ulcerations.

One of the first symptoms of ulcers is excessive hiccups. When an ulcer finally becomes noticeable, there is a searing, burning pain

1) In the stomach area just below the sternum

2) Under the rib cage on the right hand side that radiates around to the back if the ulcer is duodenal

3) In the lower bowel just below the navel if the ulcer is in the large intestine (this is called ulcerative colitis or irritable bowel).

Sometimes ulcers become so bad that they will bleed. When this happens, the stool will have red or black particles in it. The black color usually comes from bleeding in the stomach that passes through the whole intestinal tract. Bright red bleeding comes from the large intestine, or hemorrhoids. However, be aware that a stomach bleeding excessively can also cause red blood to show in the stool.

If you are prone to ulcers, become well acquainted with cayenne pepper and slippery elm. Test for and take them as often as necessary to coat the intestinal lining and promote rapid blood clotting to prevent further bleeding. Test for other herbs under "Herbs for the Stomach/Intestine" as needed to strengthen the intestinal wall. Remember to see a doctor immediately if you see any signs of blood in the stools.

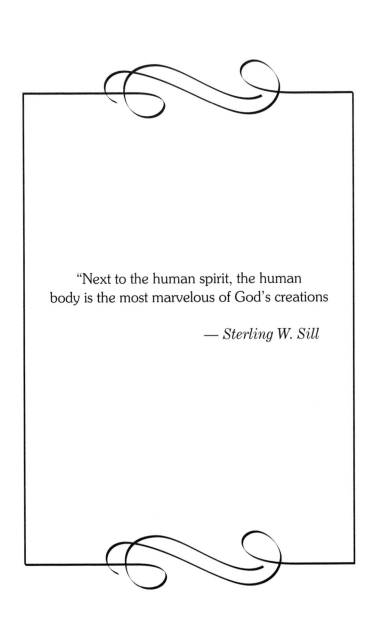

"Next to the human spirit, the human
body is the most marvelous of God's creations

— *Sterling W. Sill*

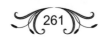

How Bio-Kinetics Helped Me . . .

Painful Stomach and Internal Distress

"Bio-Kinetics helped me where 3 physicians could not. I had painful stomach and intestinal distress accompanied by weight loss. Following the routine I needed, as discovered through the testing procedure, my problems cleared up, my pain left, and I began to gain my weight back."

> — *Jed Pitcher*
> *Chairman, CEO*
> *Blue Cross, Blue Shield*

Headaches and Acne

"I am 18 years old and have suffered from mild to severe headaches on a regular basis since early childhood. Recently my family and local doctor became very concerned and I was taken for an emergency MRI to rule out a brain tumor. Shortly thereafter I went for Bio-Kinetic testing where I discovered my problem to be parasites and Epstein-Barr Virus.

I was a typical teenager and laughed with my friends about how my "foot doctor" had figured out the cause of my headaches, but I took the herbs anyway.

I felt something different happening in my body after the first dose of herbs and decided I better take the diet and herbs seriously.

Within three days my headaches had nearly subsided. Within two weeks my acne was nearly gone. (I hadn't planned on that side benefit!) Needless to say, I'm a believer."

> — *Bryson Huckstep*
> *High School Senior*

Low Immune System—Low Energy

"Four years ago I went to my doctor to see what could be done for my low immune system and low energy. A blood test confirmed that I had the Epstein-Barr Virus. (Chronic Fatigue Syndrome)

My doctor told me nothing could be done to treat this virus and it would remain with me the rest of my life.

I continued to suffer another year until a friend with the same ailment recommended Bio-Kinetic testing. By following the program I tested for, my immune system became stronger than it was before contracting the virus and my energy levels returned to normal.

Instead of suffering through life I now have a healthy, happy life again."

> — *Robert Baxter*
> *Video Production Company Owner*
> *Winning International Arm Wrestler*

Insomnia—No Energy

"I had trouble sleeping at night, and I was tired during the day. What stressed out high school student didn't have that complaint? I had irregular menstrual cycles, but that wasn't the end of the world – my friends thought I was lucky I didn't have to worry about a period every month.

I was ornery a lot, my nerves were always just about shot, and anything could set me off, but I was under a lot of pressure in school, and I was having problems with my friends, so of course I

was upset. The most subtle, yet most substantial complaint I had was that I felt like I had never been the same since I contracted pneumonia in December of 1995.

Not only did none of these things seem substantial enough to go to a doctor, they also didn't seem to have anything in common. I ignored them and went on with my life.

I went for Bio-Kinetic testing because some of my friends had gone and I was curious to see what it was all about. I am studying medicine and wanted to see what Tisha could teach me.

She picked up on everyone of my problems, and knew their causes without me saying anything about any of them. I had Epstein Barr in various places in my body, which caused the fatigue, and the irregular menstruation. I, the queen of soft drinks, was allergic to caffeine. It hashed my nervous system and made me ornery.

The antibiotics I had taken when I had pneumonia had caused yeast to spread throughout most of my body. She put me on special cleansing diets, and gave me various herbs, and now I feel as good as new—better, because now I know how to listen to my body, and how to take care of myself."

— *Allison Hanna*
High School Student

Sick a Good Majority of the Time

"I am 29 years old and am the mother of three children. As I was growing up, I was sick a good majority of the time with colds, flu, pains and very low energy.

I sought medical help time after time and had antibiotics prescribed. I was told that the root of my illness was too much stress in my life. I could not understand this because my life was not really stressful.

I decided to accept the fact that I would never feel healthy.

My mother went for Bio-Kinetic testing seeking help for an ongoing sinus infection that the strongest antibiotics could not relieve. After doing the herbal and diet program, my mother was able to stop taking her medicine and the sinus problem was gone.

This amazed me so much that I went for an appointment.

I found out that my illness was not stress. It was Epstein-Barr and Yeast throughout my body. I got on the correct diet and herbs and within weeks I was feeling so healthy.

This was four years ago and in this time I have learned to test with Bio-Kinetics. When I feel something coming on, I know how to test and find out what is wrong and take care of the problem. I not only have been able to help myself, but my family as well.

I cannot begin to calculate the time and money Bio-Kinetics has saved me. It is so exciting to me to have more control over my own health and the health of my family."

> *— Kim Cottrell*
> *Mother*

Digestion Malfunction, Multiple Infections, Incisions That Wouldn't Heal, Shingles, Hives, Non-Existent Energy, Itched from Head to Toe

"For as long as I can remember I have had problems with digestion. They called it a nervous stomach when I was a teen. I have taken numerous anti-inflammatories and muscle relaxants, had surgery to remove spurs from the bottom of my foot, developed an esophageal reflux making it impossible to sleep without elevating my head 18—24" higher than the rest of me. I lived with hives for at least two years, had several bouts with shingles and suffered sever headaches.

I was drinking caffeine sodas for years in order to function and keep going because my energy level was non-existent. I was addicted to it. In December of 1994 I spent my Christmas recovering from a second surgery to the knee for removal of and

cartilage repair. My digestive system had almost stopped functioning.

After seven months my foot was still so painful, and the incision hadn't healed. I itched from head to toe. I had bladder and urinary infections and was getting depressed.

Through Bio-Kinetic testing I found the right diet and supplements I needed to promote healing. I had candida yeast, parasites, allergies, and Epstein-Barr.

I found that my spurs were caused by a calcium deficiency which was brought on by the medications which were beta blockers. Also, the caffeine drinks interfered with calcium absorption.

I have dissolved my spurs, my reflux has stopped, my hives have disappeared and the pain in my body has almost disappeared.

I have enjoyed doing biking and hiking without pain. What a joy it is to feel good again.

I am grateful to have learned how to do the testing so I can take charge of my own health and to help my family and others. I have come to know there are many hidden treasures of knowledge out there if we but seek them—with the Lord's help we can know if they are right for us.

I now spend four to five hours a day helping others. Life is great!!"

— Dora Tesch.,
Mother
Health and Nutritional Counselor

Depression

"The summer of 1996 was very hard for me. It was the first anniversary of my husbands death. I fell into a depressed state and became so fatigued I could not accomplish anything.

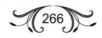

I planned my day around how many times in a day I could go up or down the stairs where the television set was. I could lay there without getting out of my pajamas, and either sleep or watch the world through the television screen.

I went to see my medical doctor and told him of my fears and concern for my health. He is a good doctor. He took blood tests and gave me a complete exam. Everything was perfectly normal.

Not wanting to continue this substandard way of life, I went for Bio-Kinetic testing. I had Epstein-Barr. After being on a program of herbs and diet changes, I began to feel better.

It wasn't long before I felt 10—20 years younger, and am enjoying a very busy energetic life again.

This good health has given me the desire to work through some life long emotional problems. I feel whole for the first time in my life."

— Carol Jones (changed for privacy)

Cancer

"I am a 68 year old female. I had three cancer surgeries and two years of chemotherapy, plus I found a new lump in my right side by the time I went for Bio-Kinetic testing. With an herbal formula, the lump disappeared in a few short weeks.

Many times with Tisha's help I have been relieved from the return of the Epstein-Barr Virus, yeast and allergies. By using the herbs and suggestions regarding diet change, etc., relief comes quickly."

— Challas Snarr
Mother, Special Education Teacher
Midvale, Utah

Allergies, Dog with a Lump, Labor and Delivery

1. "Our seven year old daughter was having a lot of allergy problems. The doctor put her on a rotation of antibiotics. Within three days of being off of them her infection would return.

We were concerned about her continued dependence on medicine, so we took her for Bio-Kinetic testing. She is now 12 years old and with the help of herbs she no longer gets infection in her sinuses.

2. Our dog had a lump the size of a baseball on his neck. The veterinarian put him on an antibiotic, and when that didn't work, he suggested exploratory surgery. My husband decided if herbs work for people, then why not try them on the dog. We gave the dog one capsule of garlic and one of cayenne pepper every morning and night wrapped in some food. Two weeks later the lump had disappeared.

3. When I was pregnant with my fourth child, I took red raspberry, along with other vitamins and herbs, the whole pregnancy. When I delivered, I had the shortest labor and easiest delivery out of all my pregnancies and I never had any afterbirth pains.

For the past five years our family has used herbs and vitamins for healing and maintenance. I feel it has kept us from catching the colds and flu that go around. When we do get sick it doesn't last. We have suffered with allergies, but as long as we stay on a maintenance of vitamins and herbs we stay healthy."

— Toni Rosander, Mother
John (Rosey) Rosander
Recreational Director

Horse Accident Causing Bruising of Body and Major Organs

"Bio-Kinetic testing and herbs have remarkably improved the health of my family over the past few years.

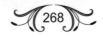

I had an incident when I fell off of a horse. On top of major bruises and some bad cuts, I found out through Bio-Kinetic testing that I had thrown most of my ribs out of place and had bruised some other organs.

I took herbs that encouraged healing, and went a few times a week to a chiropractor who confirmed the injury of my rib cage. Although I was in considerable pain, especially at night, I never spent any day in bed during this time and was able to keep up with the responsibilities of a family. I was able to avoid taking pain medication and any side effects the first week by taking Ibuprofen at night to help me sleep.

After three weeks, I felt good. This is incredible considering the injuries I sustained."

— Ursula Witzel, Mother

Migraines that Caused Passing Out

"I was 22 years old when I started getting migraines. A few months later I started passing out. As the mother of an 18 month old baby, I knew I had to do something.

I spent four months, several tests, and a lot of money on medical doctors who could not confirm a solid diagnosis.

Through Bio-Kinetic testing, taking herbs and changing my diet, within a month I was completely healthy."

— Cindy Nissalke, Mother

Feeling Run Down

"I was not feeling well. I was very run down and always tired. I went to a hospital at one time and had a four hour test run. All the results were negative. They could find nothing wrong.

I went to another doctor who diagnosed Epstein-Barr. He told me to rest and get Gamma Globulin shots every week. They told me to take it easy. Nothing got any better.

After three doctors, different results and recommendations I gave up. That was when some neighbors suggested I should try herbs. After six weeks of herbs, Bio-Kinetic testing and chiropractic visits, I was rid of Epstein-Barr. I felt much better. I could be a dad and husband again."

— Ken Carling
Computer Programmer

Fatigue

"My husband was always fatigued. He would sleep late and then feel bad that he didn't accomplish as much in the day as he wanted to. Without knowing anything about him, Bio-Kinetic testing accurately detected that he had a heart murmur and some emotional problems. After the cleansing diet there was a marked difference in his sleeping pattern. He got up earlier and had more energy in the day."

— Dilleen Marsh
School Teacher

Chronic Fatigue, Yeast, Hormonal Challenges

When I went to see Tisha, Just climbing out of the car and going up the short flight of stairs into her home created a crisis in my body. My breathing was shallow, and my heart rate was over 200 beats per minute. At that time my ankles and feet were so swollen that pants were "almost an option," not to mention that shoes were impossible to wear.

You learn to live with aches and pains, malfunctioning organs, and the results of surgeries. I found I had Epstein-Barr, parasites, yeast, allergies galore, hormonal challenges, weak thyroid, and emotional stress—all at a 10+++.

I was given herbs to take, a diet to follow, and reassurance that I would get well if I did as she instructed. It took me six weeks to cleanse and balance my body. Today I enjoy testing others and seeing my clients become well, do for themselves, and become independent.

— Lori Harrington
Mother, Spiritual Intuit

Chest Pains

"I had not been feeling well for some time. I felt extremely weak and was having chest pains and palpitations. It was exhausting to sit up in a chair. Even a piece of paper felt heavy to me. I went to several different internists who did one test after another. They could not identify the problem.

Bio-Kinetic testing revealed Epstein-Barr, yeast and allergies. I basically cut out all salt, sugar, fat, red meats, and yeast products. I took vitamins and herbs.

Initially I felt weak and had flu-like symptoms, but after a few weeks I felt such a change take place in my health. For the first time in years I had energy, my heart functioned better, and I could go walking. I was completely amazed at the change in the way I felt. The bonus in addition to feeling wonderful was that I dropped 20 pounds. Bio-Kinetics gave me back my life."

— Janis Jackson, Mother

Stomach Problems

"I am a sophomore in high school. I have had stomach problems for ten years and was always falling asleep in class. Because of this I fell behind in school, which caused me to feel depressed.

It was hard for me to follow the cleansing diet because I am a typical teenage boy, but when I did follow it, my stomach quit hurting and I began to have more energy.

I thought I would miss a month of school, but within a week I felt well enough to return to school.

As my energy increased, I became more active in school and started having great experiences with a new group of friends. I was recently voted Most Eligible Bachelor at my school and am busy and involved in school activities."

> — *Nathan Jackson*
> *High School Sophomore*

Tired and Lack of Interest

"I am a junior in high school. Two years ago I was always feeling tired and had a lack of interest in school and other activities. When I went to Tisha she found Epstein-Barr 10+++ in my body. I underwent the special diet and herbs. After one week I felt so much better and after a few more weeks I felt wonderful. I am full of energy and I've never felt better in my life."

> — *Joanna Jackson*
> *High School Junior*

Pain, Dizziness and Nausea, No Relief

"I had been having a lot of pain through my back, shoulders, and neck. Many times I'd sleep in a lazy-boy chair because I couldn't sleep on my right or left sides without feeling such excruciating pain in my shoulders and neck. It was painful to even care for my newborn. I planned one major task per day, otherwise I would be completely exhausted.

Then I developed an intense dizziness. I would lay down and the room would spin. If I got up everything would spin. Often a wave of dizziness would hit and along with it came nausea. I would throw up and have to lie down.

I was seeing a medical doctor and a chiropractor but got no answers or relief. I finally went to see Tisha. It was an incredible experience, beyond anything I had ever experienced as a nurse.

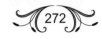

She could test me and tell me exactly what was going on in every area of my body.

Within two weeks, doing exactly as she told me, the dizziness disappeared. Within two months the lights went back on in my head and my life. My life is returned. I am able to sleep on my right and left side.

I've taken a seminar on Bio-Kinetic testing and learned the skill. Even though I am a registered nurse, I feel like someone has put a diamond in my lap and I treasure this new found knowledge. I test almost daily for myself and my family. It is invaluable. I am always learning new and valuable things."

— *Michelle Christensen*
Mother, Registered Nurse

Infertility

"My husband and I had been trying to conceive for over a year. We had one miscarriage.

We went to see Tisha because the doctors were skeptical we could get pregnant again. The procedures to get pregnant artificially were extremely costly and inconvenient—besides being improbably to work.

My husband and I both have a fast paced hectic life style. We started Tisha's program and took a few tips from her on how to slow our lives down. Within a month I conceived. Our son is now two years old and we hope to have another baby.

The medical doctors were shocked with our success. It takes time and effort to be on the herbal cleansing program but it is so worth it."

— *Cindy Jorgansen*
Businesswoman
Bryce Jorgansen
Businessman

Breast Cancer

"In March of 1997 I was diagnosed with malignant breast cancer. I was 49 years old. I agreed to radiation therapy after lumpectomy surgery. After a second surgery my surgeon and oncologist decided I needed a mastectomy. I had many doubts and negative feelings about proceeding in that direction.

My husband invited a friend who sells herbs to come and talk to me. He gave me some good advice: 'There are a lot of potential remedies out there and it can get very confusing. Don't try to do them all. Just choose one direction and stay with it.'

Another friend suggested a clinic in California that promotes a raw food diet. I felt good about going and spent three weeks there, and stayed on the diet for three months. Even before I went I felt it wasn't enough and there was still something more I needed to do.

When I returned from California, I heard about the Bio-Kinetic testing. When I went to see Tisha she seemed pleased with the herbs and diet program I had been on.

She suggested I do some mental imagery to help my body combat cancer. She told me to visualize white sheep eating grass with the sun shining behind them. The white sheep represented my white blood cells, the grass the cancer, and the sun represented God's love and healing power.

I feel the mental imagery really helped my body fight the cancer. I continue to take the herbs and supplements and was thrilled when I felt the cancer was gone. I will continue taking maintenance herbs for a year or so to stay healthy. I continue to work on boosting my immunity and helping my body be healthy.

— *Sherry Cook*
Mother

(Editors note: I recently had a visit with S.C. She had been to her medical doctor for a follow up visit and had tests run that confirmed her cancer is totally gone.)

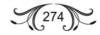

Severe Endometriosis

"I turned 30 years old this past month. I have lived a fairly active and energetic lifestyle.

In college, I met and married my best friend. After four years of not being able to conceive, I began infertility tests. These tests revealed severe endometriosis, and a hysterectomy was recommended.

Instead of the surgery, I opted for an aggressive Lupron treatment to end with inter-utero insemination in four months. The Lupron caused extensive damage to my organs.

I went for Bio-Kinetic testing which revealed Epstein-Barr, yeast "off the scale", calcium depletion, mitral valve prolapse, kidney infections, hypoglycemia, hormone imbalance (I was still in menopause from the Lupron), and weak adrenals.

Within six weeks of following the diet and herbal program, I returned for a follow up visit and felt fantastic. My eyes were clear, I had energy, my memory improved, and I had begun an exercise program. I was sleeping better at night and actually waking up with substantial energy in the mornings.

We adopted our two oldest babies shortly thereafter and I appreciated having the energy to keep up with my toddlers.

After six months on an herbal program to eliminate scar tissue, I was able to conceive a baby.

It was a difficult pregnancy and I was on bed rest a lot. We had a healthy baby boy after a difficult pregnancy and a natural posterior delivery (not intended to be normal).

My slow recovery showed just how hard the pregnancy was on my body. Medical tests revealed damage to my uterus and ovaries.

At this time I decided to make a trip to Utah for more Bio-Kinetic testing. Tisha found internal bleeding and extensive problems with

my uterus and ovaries caused from the pregnancy. My thyroid, adrenals and pancreas were all weak.

Within 24 hours of taking the herbs and vitamins suggested, I began to bleed and pass clots the size of my fist. Within two months, my uterus was no longer swelling when I'd lift my children. In six months time I was back to keeping up with my children, working out 30 minutes, and wearing size 6 clothing.

I am from a strong scientific background. My dad and uncles are all engineers, scientists, and physicians. I have found Bio-Kinetics to have an unmatched level in diagnosing and treating illness. It has been instrumental in restoring my health and has given me a new life and future wherein I can enjoy being a wife and mom."

— Julie Skalla
Mother
BA of Political Science

Appendix Index

Appendix

Epstein-Barr Cleansing Diet

1. Eliminate all foods you test allergic to.

2. Eliminate foods high in fats: red meats (pork is a red meat); deep-fried foods such as chips, french fries, donuts; thick fatty icings made from shortening or lard; high-fat dairy food like ice cream, cheese, and whole milk; Ranch, French, Blue Cheese-type dressings (use Canola or olive oil, vinegar and spices); chocolate

3. Eliminate wines and liquors; they are hard on the liver.

4. Eliminate potatoes, tomatoes, bell peppers (hot peppers are Okay), and eggplant. The Epstein-Barr virus breeds on these foods.

5. Add vitamins, minerals, and herbs that you test for.

Candida/Yeast Cleansing Diet

1. Eliminate all foods you test allergic to.

2. Eliminate all foods that are baked with bakers yeast such as breads, donuts, and pastries.

3. Eliminate foods that are aged which include cheese, wines, liquors, sour cream, blue cheese-type dressings, etc.

4. Eliminate refined sugars. Substitute raw honey, pure maple syrup, blackstrap molasses, or pineapple juice.

5. Eliminate foods that are "moldy" or "fungus-y." These include mushrooms, peanuts, peanut butter, leftovers more than two days old, etc.

6. Eliminate fruits that have a skin, high fiber content, and/or are very sweet to the taste such as apples, grapes, blueberries, pears, watermelon, strawberries, cantaloupe, etc. Citrus fruit and pineapple are acceptable if you do not test allergic to them.

7. Add vitamins, minerals, and herbs that you test for.

THINGS TO WATCH FOR IN A CLEANSE

Flu like symptoms

Sore throat

Itch, rash, skin eruptions

Frequent urination

Muscle weakness

Sleeplessness

Cramps

Fever, chills

Dizziness

Runny nose, sniffles

Loose stools

Cough

Low back ache

Depression/headache

Anxiety

Heart palpitations

Nausea, vomiting

Other

Bio-Kinetic Testing Form

BIO-KINETIC CHECKLIST

Y = Yeast   E = Epstein/Barr   P = Parasites   A = Allergies   B = Bacteria   S = Stress   M = Medicine   STD = SEXUALLY TRANSMITTED DISEASE

PHYSICAL	NOTES
Bones/Lig/Tend	
Muscles/Tissue	
Brain	
Eyes	
Ears	
Nose	
Throat	
Lungs	
Bronchial	
Heart	
Liver	
Stomach	
Small Intestine	
Large Intestine	
Nervous System	
Lymphatic System	
Spleen	
Kidneys	
Ureters	
Bladder	
Ovaries	
Uterus	
Prostate	
Blood	
Pituitary	
Thyroid	
Parathyroid	
Thymus	
Pancreas	
Adrenals	

ALLERGIES I	NOTES
Eggs	
Milk	
Wheat	
Chocolate	
Citric Acid	
Additives	
OTHER:	

ALLERGIES II	NOTES
Pesticides	
Perfumes	
Chemicals	
Gas/Diesel fumes	
Cigarette Smoke	
Pollens	
OTHER:	

The Four Rooms

Mental	
Spiritual	
Emotional	
Physical	

VITAMINS	Mg / IU	AM	NOON	PM	BED	NOTES
Vitamin A,E,D,K						
B Vitamins						
Vitamin C						
Calcium						
Multiple Vitamin						
Minerals/multiple						

HERBS	QUANTITY	AM	NOON	PM	BED	NOTES
Acid/Prima/Bifa/dophilus						
Alfalfa/Yucca						
Bilberry/Eyebright						
Black/Blue Cohosh						
Blessed Thistle/Rue						
Blue Vervain/Gotu Kola						
Brewers Yeast/AloeVera						
Buchu/Parsley						
Burdock/Yellow Dock						
Cascara/Psyllium						
Catnip/Fennel						
Cayenne/Capryllic Acid						
Chamomile/Gentian						
Cloves/Ginger						
Comfrey/Mullein						
Damiana/Dong Quai						
Dandelion/Barberry						
Dulse/Kelp						
Echinacea/Astragalus						
Essiac/Hyssop						
Eucalyptus/Horseradish						
Fatigue Drops						
Fenugreek/Thyme						
Garlic/Horehound						
Ginkgo/Hawthorn						
Ginseng/Suma						
Goldenseal/PokeRoot						
Gravel Root/Hydrange						
Irish/Iceland Moss						
Juniper/HuckleBerries						
Licorice Root/Bayberry						
Milk Thistle/Chaparral						
Mint/Horsetail						
Myrrh/Lobelia						
Nettle/Buckthorn						
Oregon Grape Root						
Pau d'Arco/Cat's Claw						
Raspberry Leaf/Fennel						
Sanicle/Cleavers						
Sarsaparilla/Sassafrass						
Saw Palmetto/FlaxSeed						
Scullcap/PassionFlower						
Slippery Elm/Chickweed						
St.John's Wort/Valerian Rt						
Uva Ursi/Marshmallow						
White Willow/White Oak						
Wild Yam/Progest Cream						
Wormwood/BlackWalnut						
Yarrow/Olive Leaf						

Suggested Reading

PHYSICAL

Back to Eden, Jethro Kloss, Woodbridge Press Publishing Company, P.O. Box 6189, Santa Barbara, CA 93111

Own Your Own Body, Stan Malstrom, Woodland Books, P.O. Box 1142, Provo, UT 84603

The Green Pharmacy, James A. Duke, PhD., Rodale Press, Emmaus, PA

Homeopathy, the Principles and Practice of Treatment, Dr. Andrew Lockie and Dr. Nicola Geddes, Houghton Mifflin Company, Boston, MA

Prescription for Nutritional Healing, James F. Balch, M.D., and Phyllis A. Balch, C.N.C, Avery Publishing Group, Inc., Garden City Park, NY

Touch For Health, John F. Thie, T.H. Enterprises, 1200 N. Lake Avenue, Pasadena, CA 91104

Hands of Light, Barbara Ann Brennan, Bantam Books

Become Younger, Norman Walker, Norwalk Press, 2218 E. Magnolia, Phoenix, AZ 85034

HerbalHome Health Care, Dr. John R. Christopher, Christopher Publications, P.O. Box 412, Springville, UT 84663

Set For Life, T Jane P. Merrill and Karen M. Sunderland, Sunrise Publishers, P.O. Box 112112, Salt Lake City, UT 84147

EMOTIONAL

Feelings Buried Alive Never Die, Karol Truman, Olympus Distributing, P.O. Box 97693, Las Vegas, NV 89193-7693

Men are from Mars, Women Are From Venus, John Gray, PhD., Harper Collins Publisher, Inc., 10 E. 53rd Street, New York, NY 10022

My Parents Married on a Dare, Carlfred Broderick, Deseret Book Company, Salt Lake City, UT

MENTAL

The Power of Positive Thinking, Norman Vincent Peale, Peale Center for Christian Living, 60 East Main Street, Pawling, NY 12564-1409

Mutant Message Down Under, Marlo Morgan, Harper Collins Publisher, Inc., 10 E. 53rd Street, New York, NY 10022

SPIRITUAL

The Book of Mormon, Church of Jesus Christ of Latter-Day Saints, Salt Lake City, UT

The Holy Bible

The Hiding Place, Corrie Ten Boom, Fleming H. Revell Company, 184 Central Avenue, Old Tappan, NJ 07675

Return from Tomorrow, George Ritchie, Baker Books

Bio-Kinetic Testing For Health
How to Take the Guesswork Out Of Healing

Seminar Information:

Tisha will be conducting seminars demonstrating the principles found in this book. The hands-on approach is always so valuable. Tisha's loving style clearly communicates so well that many have gone on to learn these skills to the point they are able to test others in the areas where they live.

I am grateful to have learned how to do the testing so I can take charge of my own health and to help my family and others. I now spend four to five hours a day helping others. Life is great!!"

— Dora Tesch., Mother
Health and Nutritional Counselor

Send all requests or questions to:

Living Dreams, LLC
PO Box 313
Sandy, UT 84091-0313

or contact Tisha at:
801-523-0890
email: tisha@aros.net

Bio-Kinetic Testing For Health
Book Order Form

❏ **YES!** I would like to get a copy(ies) of this breakthrough book teaching the skill of **Bio-Kinetic Testing For Health**. I understand *this book will help me discover these 5 secrets:*

How to save an uncalculated amount of time and money that once was used in Dr.'s offices, being sick, bills and medicines. Now it can be used towards more fun pursuits with my loved ones.

At last, what vitamins and herbs are best for my chemically unique body.

How to get control of my own personal health. I'll capture the freedom available to me because I will no longer be in the dark about what is going on with my system and what to do.

Which of the popular trends to avoid. Stop the confusion as I will be able to test and tell which ones ae right for me and which ones aren't.

When to seek medical help or when I can take care of it myself and what to do.

Send me _____ books @ $19.97 each for a total of

Shipping: _____ books @ $3.25 each for a total of

Grand Total

_____

I'll pay by: ❏ Check ❏ Money Order/Cashiers Check

(Make checks payable to *Living Dreams*, LLC)

Name_____ Phone

Address_____

City_____ State_____ Zip

Cut along this line. ✄

Fold here

Living Dreams, LLC
PO Box 313
Sandy, UT 84091-0313